Top Foods to Avoid During Your Period

Stay Healthy and Comfortable with These Simple Dietary Changes

Brenda F. Dozier

Gratitude

Dear Reader,

Thank you for choosing "Top Foods to Avoid During Your Period: Stay Healthy and Comfortable with These Simple Dietary Changes." Your decision to purchase this book is highly appreciated, and it symbolizes your dedication to bettering your health and well-being.

Writing this book has been a journey of passion and determination, inspired by the desire to provide practical, science-based counsel that empowers individuals to take charge of their menstrual health. The knowledge and ideas offered within each chapter are the result of significant research, interaction with experts, and countless hours of writing and revising. Your interest and faith in this work mean more than words can explain.

I express my gratitude to the many health professionals, researchers, and nutritionists who have given their experience and insights, helping to guarantee that the material presented is correct and beneficial. Their dedication to expanding our understanding of menstrual health has been invaluable.

To my families and friends, your reliable support and encouragement have been my anchor. Thank you for believing in this project and for your patience during the long hours spent on its production.

To you, the reader, your health and comfort during your menstrual cycle are of fundamental significance. It is my earnest desire that this book serves as a helpful guide, giving you concrete information and motivating you to make dietary adjustments that lead to increased well-being. Your journey toward better menstrual health is a personal and important one, and I am glad to be a part of it.

May the knowledge you receive from this book allow you to make educated choices that promote your health and comfort. Thank you for allowing this book to be a part of your life. Your assistance not only helps share

essential information but also inspires continued efforts
to deliver helpful resources to people who need them.

With heartfelt gratitude,

[Brenda F. Dozier].

Table of Contents

9

Introduction

The menstrual cycle is an inevitable part of life; yet, for many people, it is accompanied by a variety of unpleasant symptoms, including cramping, bloating, mood changes, and exhaustion. Millions of people face similar issues every month, and they frequently experience a sense of helplessness when confronted with the current of their bodies. On the other hand, what if I tell you that the solution to treating many of these symptoms is not found in a pill bottle but on your plate?

Welcome to "Top Foods to Avoid During Your Period: Stay Healthy and Comfortable with These Simple Dietary Changes." Your menstrual experience may be transformed via the power of smart dietary choices, and this book is your guide to making that transformation. The journey is an exploration of how the foods that we consume may either ease or intensify the symptoms that are associated with our monthly cycles. You can take charge of your menstrual health and improve your overall well-being by making strategic diet changes.

There is a important relationship between nutrition and the health of menstrual cycles. Every time we eat items that throw off our hormonal equilibrium, cause inflammation, or put a strain on our digestive system, we are inadvertently contributing to the problems that we experience throughout our menstrual cycles. This book attempts to shine a light on these hidden causes and present you with practical, science-backed options that can make your period days not just bearable but better.

Just for a moment, try to picture yourself waking up during your period feeling invigorated, with some cramping but no bloating. Picture yourself going about your everyday routines without the shadow of irritation hanging over you. This isn't a distant dream—it is a practical reality that you can reach with the appropriate dietary modifications. The things you choose to avoid might be just as potent as the ones you choose to include.

In this book, we will go deep into why some foods—like sugar, caffeine, and processed items—can be particularly difficult during your period. We will study the physiological mechanics underlying these impacts and suggest healthier options that are not only healthy for your menstrual health but also delicious and fulfilling.

This book is not simply about limitation; it is about empowerment. By understanding the influence of your food choices, you acquire the power to make decisions that support your body's natural cycles. You can minimize the intensity of your menstruation symptoms and recapture the days that might otherwise be lost to agony.

Our objective is to equip you with the information to make decisions that lead to a better, happier period. The path to enhanced menstrual health begins here, with a dedication to knowing and nourishing your body. Let this book be your trusted friend in understanding the tremendous advantages of mindful nutrition throughout your menstrual cycle. Together, we can make those hard days not just bearable but even better.

So, are you ready to start on the journey towards improved menstrual health? Are you prepared to take charge and make decisions that will lead to a better, more pleasant period? If yes, let's begin this revolutionary adventure together. Let's discover the mysteries of a menstrual-friendly diet and pave the path to a life where your period no longer controls how you feel or what you can achieve.

Together, we will investigate the top foods to avoid during your period and uncover easy, effective dietary modifications that may make a world of difference. Welcome to a new age of menstrual health—one where you are in charge.

Importance of Menstrual Health

Menstrual health is an important part of the general well-being of human beings who menstruate. It encompasses not only the physical components of the menstrual cycle but also the emotional, social, and psychological characteristics. Maintaining excellent menstrual health is crucial for various reasons, including the avoidance of reproductive health disorders, the treatment of monthly symptoms, and the increase of quality of life.

Firstly, recognizing and controlling menstrual health helps avoid numerous reproductive health disorders. Conditions such as polycystic ovarian syndrome (PCOS), endometriosis, and fibroids can greatly impair menstrual health. Early identification and careful therapy of these illnesses can avoid complications and enhance long-term health outcomes. Regular menstrual periods are frequently an indicator of hormonal balance, and any deviations might reveal underlying health concerns that require care.

Secondly, controlling menstruation symptoms correctly is crucial to preserving everyday functionality and quality of life. Menstrual health entails managing symptoms such as cramps, bloating, migraines, and mood changes. These symptoms can be burdensome for individuals, impairing their ability to conduct everyday chores, work productively, and maintain social relationships. By adopting healthy lifestyle choices, including a balanced diet, frequent exercise, and stress management skills, individuals can reduce these symptoms and enhance their overall well-being.

Furthermore, proper menstrual health is vital for mental and emotional well-being. The hormonal swings throughout the menstrual cycle might alter mood, energy levels, and cognitive performance. Understanding these shifts and using techniques to handle them can help preserve mental clarity, emotional stability, and resilience. This, in turn, develops a more optimistic attitude toward life and strengthens personal and professional connections.

Socially and culturally, menstruation health is an essential part of female equality and empowerment. Access to period hygiene products, education on menstrual health, and the removal of menstrual stigma are vital for ensuring that individuals may participate fully in all sectors of society. Promoting menstrual health and cleanliness helps break down barriers and supports the empowerment of individuals who menstruate, enabling them to pursue education, employment, and personal objectives without impediment.

Understanding Menstrual Health

Understanding menstrual health needs a holistic approach that addresses the biological, psychological, and social elements of menstruation. It entails understanding the typical phases of the menstrual cycle, evaluating variations that may suggest health difficulties, and applying activities that support good menstrual health.

Biologically, the menstrual cycle is a complicated process governed by hormone changes. It involves the interaction of the hypothalamus, pituitary gland, ovaries, and uterus. These cycle is often split into four phases: menstruation, the follicular phase, ovulation, and the luteal phase. Each phase is defined by particular hormonal changes and physiological processes that prepare the body for a prospective pregnancy.

Psychologically, menstrual health is impacted by the hormonal oscillations that occur throughout the cycle. These oscillations can influence mood, energy levels, and cognitive performance. For instance, many individuals have premenstrual syndrome (PMS), marked by symptoms such as irritability, mood swings, and anxiety, in the days leading up to menstruation. Understanding these changes can help individuals create coping skills and seek appropriate support when required.

Socially, menstruation health is impacted by cultural attitudes, access to resources, and educational opportunities. Menstrual stigma and taboos might impede individuals from accessing information and help, leading to bad health consequences. Promoting open talks about menstruation, offering access to period hygiene products, and guaranteeing complete menstrual health education are vital for building a welcoming workplace.

Effective menstrual health management entails adopting healthy lifestyle behaviors, such as keeping a balanced diet, engaging in regular physical activity, and managing stress. A diet rich in minerals, notably iron, calcium, and vitamins, helps maintain hormonal balance and alleviate menstrual discomfort. Regular exercise helps improve circulation, decrease stress, and alleviate period cramps.

Stress management practices, such as mindfulness, meditation, and deep breathing exercises, can help control hormone imbalances and promote emotional well-being.

Additionally, frequent medical check-ups are crucial for monitoring menstrual health. Healthcare practitioners can give information on managing menstruation symptoms, detecting and treating reproductive health concerns, and giving contraceptive alternatives if needed. Open conversations with healthcare professionals about menstrual health problems can lead to early discovery and appropriate management of possible difficulties.

Basics of the Menstrual Cycle

The menstrual cycle is a normal, repeating process that prepares the body for pregnancy. It usually lasts approximately 28 days; however, cycles can range from 21 to 35 days. The menstrual cycle is split into four main phases: menstruation, the follicular phase, ovulation, and the luteal phase. Each phase is defined by various hormonal changes and physiological processes.

Menstruation indicates the beginning of the menstrual cycle. It involves the loss of the uterine lining, which exits the body through the vagina as menstrual blood. Menstruation normally lasts between 3 to 7 days. The start of menstruation is initiated by a drop in the levels of estrogen and progesterone, the hormones that maintain the uterine lining.

Following menstruation is the follicular phase, which begins on the first day of menstruation and lasts until ovulation. During this period, the pituitary gland produces follicle-stimulating hormone (FSH), which encourages the formation of ovarian follicles. Each follicle carries an egg, and normally, one follicle becomes dominant and continues to grow. As the follicle matures, it generates estrogen, which helps repair the uterine lining that was destroyed during menstruation.

Ovulation happens at the midway point of the menstrual cycle, generally around day 14 of a 28-day cycle. The rise in luteinizing hormone (LH) stimulates the release of the mature egg from the dominant follicle in the ovary. The egg then proceeds down the fallopian tube, where it may contact sperm and undergo fertilization. Ovulation is the phase during the possibility of pregnancy is highest.

The luteal phase follows ovulation and lasts from roughly day 15 to day 28. After delivering the egg, the empty follicle turns into the corpus luteum, which secretes progesterone. Progesterone supports the thicker uterine lining, producing a favorable environment for a future pregnancy. If the egg is not fertilized, the corpus luteum breaks down, resulting in a reduction in progesterone levels. This hormone drop prompts the commencement of menstruation, and the cycle begins over.

Understanding the menstrual cycle is vital for detecting typical patterns and spotting any anomalies. Irregular periods, excessive bleeding, severe cramps, and other odd symptoms might signal underlying health concerns that require medical treatment. Tracking menstrual periods with a calendar or an app can help individuals monitor their cycles and spot any changes that may need further examination.

Common Symptoms and Challenges During Periods

Menstruation carries with it a range of symptoms and obstacles that might vary substantially from person to person. Understanding these symptoms and their origins can help individuals manage them more successfully and seek appropriate medical care when necessary.

One of the most frequent symptoms encountered during menstruation is menstrual cramps, commonly known as dysmenorrhea. These pains are generated by the contraction of the uterine muscles as they shed the uterine lining. Prostaglandins, hormone-like molecules, play a critical role in activating these contractions. While minor cramps are typical, severe and agonizing discomfort may suggest disorders such as endometriosis or fibroids.

Bloating and water retention are also typical during periods. Hormonal imbalances, notably the rise in estrogen, can cause the body to retain water, resulting in a sense of fullness and swelling in the belly and limbs.

Reducing salt consumption and staying hydrated can help reduce bloating.

Mood swings and emotional shifts are regularly observed throughout the menstrual cycle, particularly in the premenstrual phase. Hormonal variations, particularly changes in estrogen and progesterone levels, can impact neurotransmitter activity in the brain, influencing mood and emotional stability. Symptoms might range from irritation and anxiety to despair and exhaustion. Practicing stress management strategies and having a balanced diet can help regulate mood.

Fatigue is another typical sensation noticed with menstruation. The loss of blood can lead to a drop in iron levels, producing anemia and leading to feelings of exhaustion and poor energy. Ensuring appropriate iron intake through food or supplementation might help overcome period tiredness.

Headaches and migraines are typically connected to hormonal changes throughout the menstrual cycle. The decline in estrogen levels immediately before menstruation might produce headaches in some persons. Staying hydrated, controlling stress, and avoiding recognized triggers such as coffee and specific foods will help prevent menstrual migraines.

Digestive difficulties, including diarrhea, constipation, and nausea, can develop during menstruation. Prostaglandins, which trigger uterine contractions, can also influence the intestines, resulting in stomach pain. Eating a balanced diet rich in fiber, staying hydrated, and avoiding heavy or oily meals might help control these symptoms.

Acne and skin changes are typical throughout the menstrual cycle owing to hormonal imbalances. An increase in androgens, a kind of hormone, can encourage the sebaceous glands to generate more oil, resulting in blocked pores and breakouts. Maintaining a consistent skincare routine and avoiding harsh products can help manage menstrual acne.

Breast pain is typically reported in the days preceding menstruation. Hormonal changes, notably the rise in estrogen and progesterone, can cause the breast tissue to expand and become sensitive. Wearing a supportive bra and avoiding coffee and high-sodium meals will help minimize breast soreness.

For individuals with specific health disorders, such as PCOS, endometriosis, or fibroids, menstruation symptoms can be more intense and harder to control. PCOS is characterized by hormonal abnormalities that can lead to irregular periods, excessive hair growth, and weight gain. Endometriosis includes the development of endometrial tissue outside the uterus, producing severe discomfort and excessive bleeding. Fibroids are non-cancerous growths in the uterus that can cause excessive menstrual flow and discomfort in the pelvis. Proper diagnosis and treatment of these illnesses are critical for controlling symptoms and increasing quality of life.

In addition to physical symptoms, menstruation can bring emotional and psychological issues. The stigma and taboos around menstruation can lead to feelings of shame and humiliation, preventing individuals from seeking information and help. Addressing menstruation stigma via education and open discourse is vital for increasing menstrual health and well-being.

To treat menstruation symptoms efficiently, individuals might take several techniques. Maintaining a balanced diet rich in key minerals, such as iron, calcium, and vitamins, helps maintain hormonal balance and minimize symptoms. Regular physical exercise helps improve circulation, decrease stress, and alleviate cramps. Stress management practices, such as mindfulness, meditation, and deep breathing exercises, can help control hormone imbalances and promote emotional well-being.

Importance of Diet During Menstruation

Diet has a significant part in controlling menstrual health. During menstruation, the body undergoes major hormonal changes, and the appropriate nutritional choices can help alleviate the accompanying discomfort and symptoms. Nutrition significantly affects the body's capacity to maintain hormonal balance, manage pain, and preserve energy levels, making it crucial to pay particular attention to what we consume during this time.

One of the main reasons nutrition is crucial during menstruation is its influence on hormone control. Hormones such as estrogen and progesterone vary throughout the menstrual cycle, impacting numerous body activities. Certain meals can either help or impair the body's capacity to regulate these hormones efficiently. For example, foods rich in omega-3 fatty acids, including fish and flaxseeds, offer anti-inflammatory effects that can help regulate hormone levels and alleviate menstruation discomfort. Conversely, ingesting significant amounts of sugar and processed meals can worsen hormonal imbalances, leading to more severe symptoms.

The influence of nutrition on inflammation is another key component. Menstrual cramps are mostly caused by the creation of prostaglandins, hormone-like molecules that drive uterine muscle spasms. Foods that induce inflammation, such as those heavy in trans fats and refined carbohydrates, can increase the synthesis of prostaglandins, aggravating menstruation discomfort. In addition, anti-inflammatory foods like leafy greens, almonds, and berries can help lower inflammation and relieve cramps.

Moreover, nutrition impacts energy levels and general vitality during menstruation. The loss of blood during this period might lead to a transient decline in iron levels, resulting in weariness and weakness. Including iron-rich foods such as spinach, lentils, and lean meats will help replenish iron reserves and sustain energy levels. Additionally, complex carbs contained in whole grains and veggies give sustained energy, reducing the blood sugar rises and crashes associated with simple carbohydrates.

Proper hydration is also a critical element of nutrition during menstruation. Staying well-hydrated will help minimize bloating and relieve water retention, typical symptoms reported during periods. Drinking plenty of water and ingesting water-rich foods like cucumbers and watermelon helps support the body's hydration demands and enhance overall comfort.

Thesis Statement

By avoiding some foods and adopting simple dietary modifications, women can lessen discomfort, relieve symptoms, and enhance overall health during their period. The relationship between nutrition and period health is well-documented, with various foods known to either worsen or reduce menstruation symptoms. Implementing dietary modifications can have a tremendous influence on the physical and mental well-being of individuals during their menstrual cycle.

Avoiding foods that increase inflammation and hormonal imbalance is a significant technique for minimizing menstrual pain. Processed meals, rich in trans fats and processed carbohydrates, can stimulate the synthesis of inflammatory chemicals such as prostaglandins, leading to more severe menstrual cramps. By decreasing the intake of these items and choosing anti-inflammatory alternatives like leafy greens, almonds, and berries, individuals can drastically lower the intensity of their menstrual discomfort.

Additionally, cutting less on coffee and alcohol helps reduce typical menstruation problems. Caffeine, present in coffee, tea, and some sodas, can raise anxiety, impair sleep, and intensify menstrual cramps by constricting blood vessels. Similarly, alcohol can alter hormonal balance, dehydrate the body, and increase symptoms such as bloating and exhaustion. Replacing caffeinated and alcoholic beverages with herbal teas and water can help maintain hydration and decrease these detrimental effects.

Focusing on a nutrient-rich diet can help boost general health during menstruation. Iron-rich meals, such as spinach, lentils, and lean meats, can help counteract the weariness and weakness associated with blood loss during menstruation. Ensuring appropriate calcium intake through dairy products or plant-based substitutes can improve bone health and minimize the chance of developing osteoporosis later in life. Incorporating a range of fruits and vegetables gives critical vitamins and minerals that promote hormonal balance and general wellness.

Moreover, incorporating foods high in omega-3 fatty acids, such as fish, flaxseeds, and walnuts, helps decrease inflammation and relieve menstruation discomfort. Omega-3 fatty acids have been found to lower the formation of inflammatory prostaglandins and enhance overall cardiovascular health. These healthy fats also enhance brain function, helping to regulate mood and lessen symptoms of anxiety and despair throughout the menstrual cycle.

Managing blood sugar levels with a balanced diet is another crucial part of menstrual health. Consuming complex carbs, such as whole grains, fruits, and vegetables, gives continuous energy and reduces the blood sugar rises and crashes associated with simple carbohydrates. This helps maintain consistent energy levels and lowers cravings for sugary meals that can worsen symptoms such as bloating and mood swings.

Proper hydration is vital for treating menstruation symptoms properly. Drinking enough water helps minimize bloating, avoid dehydration, and improve general bodily functions. Consuming water-rich foods, such as cucumbers, melons, and oranges, can also aid in maintaining proper hydration levels. Avoiding high-sodium meals, which can induce water retention and exacerbate bloating, is another significant dietary modification that might enhance comfort during menstruation.

In addition to nutritional adjustments, adopting regular physical exercise can promote menstruation health. Exercise helps improve circulation, decrease stress, and lessen cramps. Activities such as yoga, swimming, and walking can be particularly useful, as they encourage relaxation and flexibility without placing excessive load on the body. Regular exercise also helps hormonal balance and general well-being, making it a crucial component of a holistic approach to menstrual health.

By making these easy dietary modifications and maintaining a healthy lifestyle, individuals can greatly lessen the discomfort and symptoms associated with menstruation. A well-balanced diet that promotes hormonal balance, decreases inflammation, and offers necessary nutrients might enhance physical and mental well-being throughout the menstrual cycle. These improvements not only increase menstruation health but also add to general health and enjoyment of life.

How Diet Can Impact Menstrual Symptoms

The relationship between nutrition and menstruation symptoms is broad and complicated. Different types of meals can alter hormonal balance, inflammation, and nutritional levels, all of which are essential variables during menstruation. Here's a summary of how nutrition might affect various menstruation symptoms:

1 Hormonal Balance:

Hormones such as estrogen and progesterone play a vital role in regulating the menstrual cycle. Certain meals can impact hormone levels and their equilibrium. For instance, increased sugar intake can lead to surges in insulin, which can influence estrogen levels and contribute to hormonal imbalances. Similarly, taking too much coffee can cause worry and stress, which in turn can alter hormone control. A diet rich in whole foods, including fruits, vegetables, lean meats, and whole grains, helps maintain stable blood sugar levels and maintains hormonal balance.

2. Inflammation:

Inflammation is a crucial element in many menstruation symptoms, notably cramps. Prostaglandins, hormone-like molecules implicated in pain and inflammation, are released in larger quantities during menstruation. Diets heavy in processed foods, refined carbohydrates, and bad fats can boost inflammation, increasing period cramps and pain. Conversely, foods rich in omega-3 fatty acids, such as fish, flaxseeds, and walnuts, have anti-inflammatory effects that can help lessen menstruation discomfort.

3. Nutrient Levels:

Menstruation leads to the loss of blood and, subsequently, important nutrients like iron. Iron deficiency can result in weariness, weakness, and anemia. Incorporating iron-rich foods such as leafy greens, beans, lentils, and lean meats will help replenish iron reserves and counteract weariness. Additionally, magnesium, found in nuts, seeds, and whole grains, is necessary for muscular relaxation and can help reduce cramps. Calcium and vitamin D are also crucial for lowering menstruation discomfort and preserving bone health.

4. Water Retention and Bloating:

High salt consumption is a major cause of water retention and bloating during menstruation. Processed meals, canned products, and salty snacks can contribute to excessive sodium consumption, worsening these symptoms. Reducing salt consumption and staying hydrated by drinking enough of water can help reduce bloating. Including potassium-rich foods, such as bananas, avocados, and sweet potatoes, can also help regulate salt levels and prevent water retention.

5. Digestive Health:

Digestive difficulties, such as constipation or diarrhea, are frequent during menstruation owing to hormonal variations influencing gut motility. A diet high in fiber, including fruits, vegetables, and whole grains, supports good digestion and can help reduce these symptoms. Additionally, probiotics contained in yogurt and fermented foods like kimchi and sauerkraut support healthy gut microbiota, which can benefit overall digestive health.

6. Mental and Emotional Well-Being:

The emotional and psychological components of menstruation are impacted by nutrition as well. Serotonin, a neurotransmitter that affects mood, is altered by the foods we eat. Consuming complex carbs, such as whole grains and legumes, can enhance serotonin levels and improve mood. Omega-3 fatty acids also boost brain function and can help alleviate anxiety and despair. Avoiding excessive coffee and sugar, which can contribute to mood swings and impatience, is vital for maintaining emotional stability during menstruation.

Brief Overview of the Book's Purpose

This book, "Top Foods to Avoid During Your Period: Stay Healthy and Comfortable with These Simple Dietary Changes," is aimed to give detailed counsel on how dietary choices might impact menstrual health. The objective of this book is to educate and empower women to make educated decisions regarding their food during menstruation, helping them reduce common symptoms and boost their general health and well-being.

Menstrual health is a complicated interaction of different elements, with food being a crucial one. While medical therapies and lifestyle modifications play essential roles, the foods ingested can either relieve or increase menstruation symptoms. This book tries to bridge the gap between scientific understanding and practical application, presenting concrete advice that may be easily adopted into daily life.

The book opens with a discussion of the importance of menstrual health, highlighting why it should be a priority for individuals who menstruate. Understanding the principles of the menstrual cycle and understanding typical symptoms and issues gives a basis for grasping the influence of nutrition on menstrual health. Each chapter digs into particular foods that should be avoided, detailing the scientific reasons behind their adverse impact on menstrual health. It also gives healthier options and practical recommendations for making dietary adjustments that might lead to a more comfortable and managed menstruation experience.

This book offers a thorough guide for women looking to enhance their menstrual health via informed food choices. By understanding the importance of nutrition in managing menstruation symptoms, women may take proactive actions to lessen discomfort, increase their well-being, and maintain a healthy lifestyle throughout their menstrual cycle.

Chapter 1

The Connection Between Diet and Menstrual Health

The relationship between nutrition and menstruation health is broad and complicated. What we consume greatly affects our hormonal balance, the intensity of menstruation symptoms, and general reproductive health. Understanding this relationship can empower individuals to adopt dietary choices that support a healthier menstrual cycle and alleviate common difficulties connected with menstruation.

Our bodies rely on a precise balance of hormones to control the menstrual cycle. Hormones including estrogen, progesterone, and insulin are all regulated by the meals we consume. A diet strong in processed sweets and bad fats can upset this equilibrium, resulting in more severe menstruation symptoms. Conversely, a diet rich in whole foods, healthy fats, and necessary nutrients can enhance hormonal equilibrium and alleviate pain.

Moreover, the inflammatory response in the body, which is directly connected to nutrition, plays a vital part in the experience of menstruation symptoms. meals that increase inflammation, such as processed meals and those high in trans fats, can worsen problems like cramping and bloating. On the other side, anti-inflammatory meals, notably those high in omega-3 fatty acids, can help reduce these symptoms.

The nutritious quality of our food also influences menstruation health. Nutrient deficiencies can contribute to a range of concerns, from increased tiredness and mood fluctuations to more significant reproductive health problems. Ensuring a diet that contains appropriate vitamins and minerals is vital for maintaining energy levels, lowering stress, and boosting the body's capacity to cope with the demands of the menstrual cycle.

How Diet Affects Menstrual Symptoms

Diet has a direct influence on the degree and kind of menstruation symptoms experienced. Understanding how different meals influence the body during menstruation might help individuals manage their symptoms more efficiently.

1. Menstrual Cramps:

Menstrual cramps are one of the most prevalent and uncomfortable sensations encountered during menstruation. These pains are triggered by the production of prostaglandins, which are hormone-like molecules that drive uterine contractions. Certain meals can alter the generation of prostaglandins and the intensity of cramps. Diets heavy in processed foods, refined carbohydrates, and unhealthy fats can promote inflammation and the synthesis of prostaglandins, leading to more acute cramps. Conversely, ingesting foods high in anti-inflammatory characteristics, such as leafy greens, berries, and fatty fish, can help minimize the intensity of cramps.

2. Bloating and Water Retention:

Bloating and water retention are frequent problems during menstruation, generally caused by hormonal changes that disrupt fluid balance in the body. High salt consumption is a primary contributor to water retention, as it leads the body to hold onto surplus fluid. Processed meals and salty snacks are often rich in sodium and should be reduced during menstruation. Instead, ingesting potassium-rich foods like bananas, avocados, and sweet potatoes can help regulate salt levels and prevent bloating. Staying well-hydrated by consuming enough water also assists in reducing water retention.

3. Mood Swings and Emotional Changes:

Hormonal variations throughout the menstrual cycle can contribute to mood swings, anxiety, and sadness. Diet can play a crucial role in treating these emotional problems. Consuming complex carbs, such as whole grains, legumes, and fruits, helps maintain steady blood sugar levels, which can stabilize mood. Omega-3 fatty acids, found in foods like salmon, flaxseeds, and walnuts, are also excellent for brain function and can help alleviate anxiety and sadness. Additionally, avoiding excessive coffee and sugar, which can create spikes and falls in blood sugar levels, might assist in maintaining emotional equilibrium.

4. Fatigue:

Fatigue is a frequent symptom during menstruation, often related to the loss of blood and the consequent fall in iron levels. Iron deficiency can lead to anemia, marked by tiredness, weakness, and trouble focusing. Consuming iron-rich foods, such as lean meats, leafy greens, beans, and fortified cereals, can aid to restore iron reserves and counteract weariness. Pairing these meals with sources of vitamin C, such as citrus fruits and bell peppers, improves iron absorption. Ensuring proper consumption of additional energy-boosting nutrients, such as B vitamins and magnesium, is also vital for sustaining energy levels during menstruation.

5. Headaches and Migraines:

Many individuals get headaches and migraines around the time of their period, sometimes prompted by hormonal imbalances. Estrogen levels decline right before menstruation, which can cause headaches. Diet can influence the frequency and intensity of these headaches. For example, dehydration is a typical cause of headaches, so staying hydrated is vital. Certain foods, such as those containing tyramine (found in old cheeses and processed meats), can also provoke migraines and should be avoided by people prone to monthly headaches. Including magnesium-rich foods, such as nuts, seeds, and dark chocolate, can help avoid migraines, as magnesium plays a role in nerve activity and blood flow.

Hormonal Balance and Diet

Maintaining hormonal balance is vital for a healthy menstrual cycle, and nutrition plays a key part in this process. Hormones are chemical messengers that govern numerous biological activities, including the menstrual cycle. The balance of hormones such as estrogen, progesterone, insulin, and cortisol can be changed by the foods we consume.

1. Estrogen and Progesterone:

Estrogen and progesterone are the major hormones controlling the menstrual cycle. An imbalance in these hormones can lead to irregular periods, excessive bleeding, and severe PMS symptoms. Phytoestrogens, plant substances that mimic estrogen in the body, can help regulate estrogen levels. Food's high in phytoestrogens include soy products, flaxseeds, and legumes. Additionally, cruciferous vegetables like broccoli, cauliflower, and Brussels sprouts have chemicals that assist the body absorb estrogen more effectively, supporting hormonal balance.

2. Insulin:

Insulin is a hormone which controls blood sugar levels. Diets heavy in refined sugars and simple carbs can lead to insulin resistance, which can disturb hormonal balance and contribute to illnesses like polycystic ovarian syndrome (PCOS). Consuming complex carbs, such as whole grains and legumes, helps maintain stable blood sugar levels and improves insulin sensitivity. Including protein and healthy fats in meals also helps manage blood sugar and insulin levels.

3. Cortisol:

Cortisol, the stress hormone, can influence the menstrual cycle when levels are continuously increased. Stress and poor dietary choices, such as ingesting too much coffee and sugar, can boost cortisol levels. High cortisol can disturb the balance of other hormones, leading to irregular periods and increased PMS symptoms. Managing stress with healthy lifestyle choices, such as frequent physical activity, appropriate sleep, and a balanced diet, can help manage cortisol levels. Foods high in antioxidants, such as berries and leafy greens, can also help alleviate the effects of stress on the body.

4. Thyroid Hormones:

Thyroid hormones control metabolism and have a role in menstrual health. An underactive thyroid (hypothyroidism) can contribute to irregular periods, excessive bleeding, and exhaustion. Ensuring appropriate consumption of minerals that promote thyroid function, such as iodine (found in seafood and iodized salt), selenium (found in Brazil nuts and seafood), and zinc (found in meat and seeds), is vital for maintaining hormonal balance.

Nutrient Deficiencies and Their Impact

Nutrient deficiencies can have a substantial influence on menstruation health, leading to a range of symptoms and consequences. Ensuring proper consumption of vital vitamins and minerals is crucial for maintaining a healthy menstrual cycle and reducing typical menstruation symptoms.

1. Iron:

Iron insufficiency is a typical concern for persons with excessive menstrual flow. Iron is important for creating hemoglobin, the protein in red blood cells that delivers oxygen throughout the body. A deficiency can lead to anemia, marked by weariness, weakness, and shortness of breath. Consuming iron-rich foods, such as lean meats, beans, lentils, and leafy greens, helps rebuild iron reserves. Pairing these meals with sources of vitamin C, such as citrus fruits, improves iron absorption.

2. Magnesium:

Magnesium is a mineral that has a role in muscle relaxation and nerve function. It is particularly beneficial for reducing menstrual cramps and avoiding migraines. Magnesium insufficiency can lead to increased muscular tension and cramps. Food's high in magnesium which consist of nuts, seeds, whole grains, and dark leafy greens. Including these items in the diet can help minimize the intensity of period cramps and migraines.

3. Calcium:

Calcium is vital for keeping strong bones and minimizing menstruation discomfort. It helps control muscle contractions, particularly those in the uterus. A calcium deficit can contribute to greater muscular cramps and discomfort during menstruation. Dairy products, fortified plant-based milks, and leafy greens are rich sources of calcium. Ensuring proper intake of calcium can help reduce period cramps and improve overall bone health.

4. Vitamin D:

Vitamin D serves a function in regulating the menstrual cycle and decreasing inflammation. A lack of vitamin D can lead to hormonal abnormalities and raise the risk of illnesses like PCOS. Vitamin D is generated in the skin through exposure to sunshine, but it may also be taken from foods such as fatty fish, fortified dairy products, and egg yolks. Adequate vitamin D levels support hormonal balance and minimize menstruation symptoms.

5. B Vitamins:

B vitamins, notably B6 and B12, are vital for energy generation and mood control. They have a role in the creation of neurotransmitters, which impact mood and cognitive function. Deficiencies in B vitamins can contribute to weariness, sadness, and irritability during menstruation. Foods high in B vitamins include entire grains, lean meats, eggs, and dairy products. Ensuring appropriate consumption of these vitamins can assist in maintaining energy levels and emotional stability.

6. Omega-3 Fatty Acids:

Omega-3 fatty acids contain anti-inflammatory qualities that can help lessen menstruation discomfort and enhance mood. A deficit in omega-3s might contribute to increased inflammation and worsening menstruation symptoms. Food's high in omega-3 fatty acids include fatty fish, flaxseeds, chia seeds, and walnuts. Including these items in the diet can help decrease inflammation and relieve period cramps.

The Science Behind Food Choices

Understanding the science behind dietary choices during the menstrual cycle can dramatically increase menstrual health. The minerals and chemicals in diverse meals interact with the body in ways that can either reduce or intensify menstruation symptoms. The link between nutrition and menstrual health involves complicated biochemical processes, including hormone control, inflammation, and nutrient absorption.

Hormones like estrogen and progesterone change throughout the menstrual cycle, impacting how the body responds to different diets. For example, certain meals can improve the liver's capacity to metabolize estrogen, while others can encourage the creation of progesterone. Additionally, the inflammatory response in the body, which may be altered by nutrition, plays a key role in menstruation symptoms such as cramps and bloating.

Understanding these biochemical relationships can help individuals make educated food decisions that promote menstrual health.

Research on Diet and Menstrual Health

Research has demonstrated that nutrition has a key influence on menstrual health. Various research has studied the influence of certain nutrients and dietary patterns on menstruation symptoms and overall reproductive health.

One prominent field of study is the role of anti-inflammatory diets. For instance, a study published in the American Journal of Clinical Nutrition found that women who consumed diets high in anti-inflammatory foods, such as fruits, vegetables, and omega-3 fatty acids, experienced fewer menstrual symptoms compared to those with diets high in processed foods and unhealthy fats. The anti-inflammatory effects of these foods help lower the synthesis of prostaglandins, which are connected with menstruation cramps and inflammation.

Another field of study explores the influence of micronutrients on menstrual health. Studies have emphasized the role of iron, magnesium, calcium, and vitamin D in regulating menstruation discomfort. For example, a study published in The Journal of Nutrition indicated that appropriate consumption of magnesium can help lessen the severity of menstrual cramps, while sufficient iron intake is critical for avoiding anemia and exhaustion associated with heavy monthly flow.

Additionally, research on hormonal balancing has revealed that diets high in fiber can help control estrogen levels. Research in The Lancet found that women who consumed larger quantities of dietary fiber had lower levels of circulating estrogen, which can help reduce the risk of estrogen-related illnesses such as breast cancer and endometriosis.

The Healthiest Foods to Eat During Every Phase of Your Monthly Cycle

The menstrual cycle contains of four main phases: the menstrual phase, the follicular phase, the ovulatory phase, and the luteal phase. Each phase has distinct hormonal changes that may be supported by certain meals to maximize health and ease discomfort.

1. Menstrual Phase (Days 1-5):

During the menstrual period, the body loses the uterine lining, resulting in blood loss and a drop in energy levels. It is vital to focus on nutrient-dense meals that assist replace lost iron and promote overall energy.

Iron-rich foods: Spinach, lean red meat, lentils, and fortified cereals.

Anti-inflammatory foods: Berries, tomatoes, and fatty seafood like salmon.

Hydrating foods: Cucumbers, watermelon, and citrus fruits.

Energy-boosting foods: Whole grains, nuts, and seeds.

2. Follicular Phase (Days 6-14):

The follicular phase involves the development of follicles in the ovaries, leading up to ovulation. Estrogen levels begin to rise, which can be supported by meals that promote good estrogen metabolism and overall energy.

Phytoestrogen are foods that are rich foods: Soy products, flaxseeds, and sesame seeds.

Protein-rich foods: Eggs, poultry, and lentils.

Folate-rich foods: Leafy greens, avocados, and legumes.

Complex simple carbohydrate: Quinoa, brown rice, and sweet potatoes.

3. Ovulatory Phase (Days 15-17):

Through the ovulatory phase, an egg is released from the ovary. This period is distinguished by a surge in estrogen and luteinizing hormone (LH). Nutrient-dense diets that maintain hormone balance and give prolonged energy are advantageous.

Antioxidant-rich foods: Blueberries, cherries, and dark chocolate.

Healthy fats: Avocados, olive oil, and almonds.

Zinc-rich foods: Pumpkin seeds, chickpeas, and cashews.

Fiber-rich foods: Whole grains, fruits, and vegetables.

4. Luteal Phase (Days 18-28):

The luteal phase is marked by a surge in progesterone, preparing the body for a prospective pregnancy. Many women have premenstrual syndrome (PMS) during this time, including symptoms including bloating, mood swings, and cravings.

Magnesium-rich foods: Bananas, dark leafy vegetables, and dark chocolate.

Calcium-rich foods: Yogurt, cheese, and almonds.

B6-rich foods: Sunflower seeds, pistachios, and poultry.

Complex carbohydrates: Oats, barley, and sweet potatoes.

Hydrating foods: Cucumbers, celery, and water-rich fruits.

What to Eat During Each Stage of Your Menstrual Cycle?

Dietary choices may be adapted to each stage of the menstrual cycle to enhance health and ease discomfort. Here's a full guidance on what to eat at each stage:

Menstrual Phase (Days 1-5):

During menstruation, the focus should be on restoring lost nutrients and controlling symptoms like cramping and exhaustion.

Breakfast: A smoothie with spinach, cherries, Greek yogurt, and chia seeds.

Lunch: A salad with mixed greens, grilled chicken, quinoa, and a citrus vinaigrette.

Snack: Almonds and an apple.

Dinner: Lentil soup with a side of whole-grain bread.

Hydration: Herbal teas (such as chamomile or ginger) and lots of water.

Follicular Phase (Days 6-14):

In the follicular phase, the focus is on sustaining estrogen production and supplying energy for the active development of follicles.

Breakfast: Oatmeal topped with flaxseeds, berries, and a sprinkle of honey.

Lunch: A quinoa dish with black beans, corn, avocado, and salsa.

Snack: Carrot sticks with hummus.

Dinner: Baked salmon with a side of roasted Brussels sprouts and brown rice.

Hydration: Green tea and infused water with lemon and mint.

Ovulatory Phase (Days 15-17):

During ovulation, nutrient-rich meals that promote energy and antioxidant consumption are good.

Breakfast: Greek yogurt with blueberries, walnuts, and a sprinkling of cinnamon.

Lunch: A spinach and strawberry salad with goat cheese and balsamic dressing.

Snack: A handful of mixed nuts.

Dinner: Grilled chicken with a side of quinoa and roasted veggies.

Hydration: Pomegranate juice and plenty of water.

Luteal Phase (Days 18-28):

In the luteal phase, the focus is on treating PMS symptoms and promoting progesterone production.

Breakfast: A bowl of enriched cereal with almond milk and sliced bananas.

Lunch: A wrap with turkey, avocado, spinach, and whole-grain tortilla.

Snack: Dark chocolate and a handful of sunflower seeds.

Dinner: Stir-fry with tofu, broccoli, bell peppers, and brown rice.

Hydration: Chamomile tea and plenty of water.

Expert Opinions and Case Studies

Expert perspectives and case studies give significant insights into how food choices might impact menstrual health. Nutritionists, dietitians, and healthcare experts have long argued for the significance of nutrition in controlling menstruation symptoms and boosting general well-being.

Expert Opinions:

Dr. Mary Jane Minkin, a clinical professor of obstetrics, gynecology, and reproductive sciences at Yale University, highpoints the importance of food in menstruation health. She adds that including anti-inflammatory foods, such as omega-3 fatty acids and antioxidants, might help minimize period discomfort and inflammation. Dr. Minkin also underlines the benefits of magnesium for muscular relaxation and calcium for alleviating menstrual cramps.

Registered dietitian Alissa Rumsey, MS, RD, says that a balanced diet rich in whole foods can help regulate hormones and ease PMS symptoms. She suggests focusing on fiber-rich meals to promote estrogen metabolism and decrease bloating. Rumsey also suggests staying hydrated and avoiding coffee and alcohol intake, since these might increase menstruation symptoms.

Case Studies:

Case studies present real-world examples of how dietary modifications might enhance menstrual health. One significant example includes a 32-year-old lady having severe PMS symptoms, including mood swings, bloating, and cramps. After consulting with a qualified dietitian, she undertook dietary modifications such as eliminating refined carbohydrates, increasing her consumption of leafy greens and omega-3 fatty acids, and integrating magnesium-rich foods. Within three months, she reported a dramatic reduction in her PMS symptoms and an overall increase in her energy levels and happiness.

Another case study concerns a 28-year-old lady with excessive menstrual flow and iron deficiency anemia. After modifying her diet to include more iron-rich foods, such as lean meats, lentils, and spinach, and mixing them with vitamin C-rich meals for enhanced absorption, she saw a decrease in fatigue and an increase in her general health. Her iron levels normalized, and her excessive bleeding became fairly bearable.

The relationship between nutrition and menstruation health is clear via scientific research, professional perspectives, and real-world case studies. Understanding the science underlying food choices and their influence on menstruation symptoms can empower individuals to make educated dietary decisions. By including nutrient-dense, anti-inflammatory, and hormone-supportive foods in their diet, individuals may maximize their menstrual health and decrease typical symptoms linked with the menstrual cycle.

Chapter 2

Smart food choices

Understanding the function of particular foods in regulating menstrual health can lead to better results and enhanced well-being. Here are thorough insights into many essential dietary types and their advantages during menstruation.

Water-Rich Fruits: Hydration and Natural Sweetness

Water-rich fruits like watermelon and cucumber are wonderful alternatives for hydration and give natural sweetness without the additional sugars found in processed foods. These fruits not only assist in maintaining fluid balance but also offer a spectrum of nutrients that can improve general health during menstruation.

Watermelon: This fruit is made up of almost 90% water, making it a perfect choice for staying hydrated.

Hydration is vital during menstruation as it helps to decrease bloating and can lower the severity of cramping. Watermelon is also an excellent source of vitamins A and C, which are antioxidants that help protect cells from harm and strengthen the immune system.

Cucumber: Like watermelon, cucumbers have a high-water content, it helps to keep the body hydrated. Cucumbers are also low in calories and rich in vitamins K and B, as well as minerals like magnesium and potassium. These nutrients aid in maintaining good blood pressure and muscular function, which might be advantageous during periods when cramps are prevalent.

Incorporating water-rich fruits into the diet may be simple and fun. For example, a pleasant watermelon and cucumber salad with a dash of lime juice may be a hydrated and nutritious snack. Additionally, adding slices of these fruits to water might make hydration more enticing and tastier.

Leafy Green Vegetables: Boosting Iron Levels and Combating Fatigue

Leafy green vegetables such as kale and spinach are nutritional powerhouses that can considerably boost menstrual health. These greens are high in iron, a key element that helps battle the exhaustion frequently associated with menstruation, especially in individuals with heavy periods.

Kale: Kale is a nutrient-dense vegetable that supplies a large quantity of iron, which is required for the formation of hemoglobin in red blood cells. Adequate iron levels help prevent anemia, a disorder marked by tiredness and weakness. Kale is also rich in vitamin K, which is vital for blood clotting and bone health, and vitamin C, which increases iron absorption.

Spinach: Spinach is other good source of iron, particularly non-heme iron, which is present in plant-based meals. To increase iron absorption, it's helpful to match spinach with vitamin C-rich meals. Spinach is also abundant in folate, a B vitamin that encourages the development of new cells, and magnesium, which can help ease period cramps by relaxing muscles.

Combining leafy greens into dishes may be straightforward and flexible. A spinach and kale smoothie, for instance, can be a healthful way to start the day. Additionally, adding these greens to soups, stews, and salads will help ensure a proper intake of these important elements.

Ginger: Anti-Inflammatory Effects and Nausea Relief

Ginger is a well-known natural treatment with significant anti-inflammatory effects and the capacity to ease nausea, making it a great addition to the diet during menstruation.

Anti-Inflammatory benefits: Ginger includes bioactive chemicals including gingerol, which have potent anti-inflammatory and antioxidant benefits. These characteristics can help lessen menstrual pain and cramps by reducing the synthesis of prostaglandins, substances in the body that produce inflammation and discomfort. Several studies have indicated that ginger can be as beneficial as non-steroidal anti-inflammatory medicines (NSAIDs) in lowering menstruation discomfort.

Nausea Relief: Ginger is also useful in reducing nausea, which some women feel throughout their menstrual cycle. The chemical components in ginger aid in promoting digestive reactivity and speed up the emptying of the stomach, which helps alleviate symptoms of nausea.

Ginger into the diet may be done in numerous ways. Fresh ginger tea, produced by steeping sliced ginger in hot water, may be calming and healthful. Adding grated ginger to smoothies, stir-fries, or soups can also boost flavor and give health benefits.

Protein-Rich Foods: Curbing Cravings and Supporting Overall Health

Protein-rich meals such as chicken and fish have a critical role in reducing cravings and boosting overall health during menstruation. Protein helps to balance blood sugar levels, which can avoid the extreme cravings for sweet and high-fat meals that many women experience during their period.

Chicken: Chicken is a fantastic source of lean protein, in which helps to retain muscle mass and repair tissues. It also includes crucial minerals including B vitamins, which are essential for energy generation and lowering weariness. The high protein level in chicken can help keep you satisfied for longer, minimizing the chance of harmful snacking.

Fish: Fish, particularly fatty fish like salmon, is rich in omega-3 fatty acids, which have anti-inflammatory qualities. Omega-3s can help lessen menstruation discomfort and inflammation. Fish is also a strong source of vitamin D, which has been found to help regulate mood and lower the risk of depression, a typical symptom associated with PMS.

Protein-rich foods into the diet may be done through easy and delightful meals. Grilled chicken breasts with a side of veggies or a salmon fillet with a quinoa salad are healthful alternatives that supply high-quality protein and important elements.

Turmeric: Anti-Inflammatory Spice with Curcumin

Turmeric, a brilliant yellow spice often used in Indian cuisine, includes curcumin, a molecule with significant anti-inflammatory effects. Including turmeric in the diet can give various benefits for menstrual health.

Anti-Inflammatory Properties: Curcumin, the main element in turmeric, has been widely investigated for its anti-inflammatory benefits. It acts by reducing the function of inflammatory substances in the body, including cytokines and enzymes like cyclooxygenase-2 (COX-2). This can help reduce period pain and inflammation, similar to how NSAIDs work but without the associated negative effects.

Pain Relief: Research has indicated that curcumin can be useful in lowering the intensity of menstruation pain. Research published in the Journal of Family & Reproductive Health revealed that women who took curcumin supplements saw substantial decreases in PMS symptoms, including mood swings, discomfort, and bloating.

Integrating turmeric into the diet may be both fun and useful. Adding turmeric to soups, stews, and curries can increase flavor and give health benefits. Golden milk, a traditional Indian drink prepared with turmeric, milk, and other spices, may be a calming beverage that helps decrease inflammation and enhance general health.

Practical Tips for Including These Foods in Your Diet (continued)

Hydration with Water-Rich Fruits: Incorporate watermelon and cucumber into your everyday snacks or meals. A watermelon and feta cheese salad may be a delicious and hydrating alternative. Similarly, cucumber slices with hummus make for a healthful and hydrated snack.

Leafy Green Vegetables: Add kale and spinach to your smoothies, salads, and main meals. A green smoothie with spinach, kale, banana, and almond milk may be a healthful start to your day. For lunch or supper, a quinoa and kale salad with roasted veggies and a lemon-tahini dressing can be both filling and nutrient-dense.

Ginger for Anti-Inflammatory and Nausea Relief: Make ginger tea by steeping fresh ginger slices in boiling water. This can be eaten throughout the day to assist control of menstruation pain. Additionally, adding ginger to stir-fries, soups, and marinades can enhance the flavor and bring health benefits.

Protein-Rich Foods: Include a range of protein sources in your meals. Grilled chicken breast with a side of roasted veggies or a salmon fillet with a quinoa and avocado salad are perfect alternatives. For vegans, lentils, chickpeas, and tofu can be wonderful protein-rich options.

Turmeric as an Anti-Inflammatory Spice: Add turmeric to your recipes to improve their nutritional content. Turmeric may be used in rice, soups, and stews for a rich color and health benefits. Golden milk, prepared with turmeric, milk, honey, and a dash of black pepper, may be a pleasant beverage that enhances menstrual health.

By knowing the science behind these smart food choices and adding them to your diet, you can support your menstrual health and general well-being. Making simple, educated adjustments to your diet can lead to big gains in controlling menstruation symptoms and boosting your quality of life.

Best Foods to Eat During Your Period and Other Reproductive Tips

Eating the appropriate meals during menstruation can substantially affect how you feel and manage symptoms. Here are some of the healthiest things to incorporate into your diet during your period:

1. Dark Leafy Greens: Vegetables like spinach, kale, and Swiss chard are high in iron, which helps restore the iron lost via menstrual blood. Iron is vital for maintaining energy levels and reducing exhaustion during your period.

2. Fatty Fish: Salmon, mackerel, and sardines are great providers of omega-3 fatty acids, which have anti-inflammatory qualities. Omega-3s can help reduce period cramps and inflammation, making these fish ideal additions to your diet.

3. Nuts and Seeds: Almonds, walnuts, chia seeds, and flaxseeds are rich in dynamic fatty acids, magnesium, and vitamin E. These nutrients can help reduce bloating, control mood swings, and maintain overall hormonal balance.

4. Whole Grains: Whole grains including brown rice, quinoa, oats, and barley contain complex carbs that deliver energy slowly. This helps balance blood sugar levels and lowers cravings for sugary meals that might cause mood swings.

5. Lean Protein: Chicken, turkey, tofu, and lentils are rich sources of protein that help balance blood sugar levels and improve muscle health. Protein-rich diets can help reduce cravings and enhance serotonin levels, enhancing mood and lowering irritation.

6. Yogurt: Opt for plain yogurt with living cultures to enhance digestive health. Yogurt is a strong source of calcium and vitamin D, which can help minimize PMS symptoms such as bloating and mood swings.

7. Bananas: Bananas are rich in potassium, which helps maintain fluid balance in the body and minimizes water retention and bloating. They also include vitamin B6, which can help reduce premenstrual symptoms.

8. Herbal Teas: Chamomile tea and peppermint tea are recognized for their relaxing properties and can help lessen period cramps and encourage relaxation.

In addition to including these items in your diet, consider following reproductive health tips:

Stay Hydrated: Drink lots of water to maintain hydration levels, which is vital for general health and symptom management during menstruation.

Exercise Regularly: Engage in light to moderate exercise, such as walking, yoga, or swimming, to improve circulation, decrease stress, and alleviate period cramps.

Manage Stress: Practice stress-reducing practices like deep breathing, meditation, or journaling to lessen the influence of stress on menstruation symptoms.

Get Adequate Sleep: Aim for 7-9 hours of quality sleep every night to promote hormone homeostasis and general well-being.

Top 3 Spices to Help Relieve PMS Symptoms Recommended by an Expert

Spices have been used for ages to ease different health conditions, including menstruation cramps. Here are three spices recommended by professionals for treating PMS symptoms:

1. Ginger: Ginger is recognized for its anti-inflammatory effects and can help alleviate period cramps and nausea. It also improves digestion and can decrease bloating linked with PMS. Fresh ginger may be soaked in hot water to produce ginger tea or added to smoothies, soups, and stir-fries.

2. Turmeric: Turmeric contains curcumin, a potent antioxidant and anti-inflammatory substance. Curcumin helps decrease inflammation and discomfort linked with menstrual cramps. Turmeric can be added to curries, soups, or golden milk (turmeric latte) for its health advantages.

3. Cinnamon: Cinnamon has been demonstrated to help regulate menstrual periods and minimize excessive bleeding. It as well contains anti-inflammatory effects that can help reduce cramps and bloating. Sprinkle cinnamon on porridge, or yogurt, or add it to smoothies and baked goods for a warming and soothing flavor.

These spices not only provide taste to recipes but also give natural solutions for treating PMS symptoms. Incorporating them into your diet can enhance overall menstrual health and relieve pain.

The Significance of Staying Hydrated During Your Period

Staying hydrated is vital for general health and well-being, especially during menstruation. Here's why hydration matters:

1. Fluid Balance: Drinking a proper amount of water helps maintain fluid balance in the body. This is vital during menstruation, as hormonal changes can contribute to fluid retention and bloating. Proper water can help ease these symptoms.

2. Temperature Regulation: Hydration improves the body's capacity to control temperature, which might fluctuate during menstruation. Proper hydration helps avoid overheating or excessive cold sensitivity.

3. Nutrient Transport: Water is necessary for delivering nutrients throughout the body, especially to cells and tissues involved in reproductive health. It ensures that important nutrients reach their appropriate destinations, promoting overall menstrual health.

4. Waste Removal: Adequate water improves kidney function and helps flush out toxins and waste products from the body. This can minimize the incidence of urinary tract infections (UTIs) and help overall detoxification.

How Water Reduces Bloating and Prevents Dehydration Headaches

Water serves a significant function in minimizing bloating and avoiding dehydration headaches during menstruation:

1. Reducing Bloating: Drinking water helps flush away extra salt and waste materials that can lead to bloating. It also improves digestive health by assisting in the flow of food and waste through the gastrointestinal system, decreasing constipation and bloating.

2. Preventing Dehydration Headaches: Dehydration can contribute to headaches and migraines, which can be aggravated during menstruation owing to hormonal changes. Drinking enough water helps maintain optimum hydration levels, minimizing the incidence of dehydration headaches.

3. Alleviating Cramps: Proper hydration can help reduce muscular cramps, especially menstrual cramps, by providing appropriate blood flow and oxygen delivery to muscles. This can lower the intensity and length of cramps, increasing overall comfort during menstruation.

4. Improving Mood and Energy Levels: Dehydration can contribute to feelings of weariness and irritation, which are prevalent during menstruation. Drinking water helps sustain energy levels and maintains mood stability, supporting overall well-being.

Chapter 3

Foods to Avoid: Sugar and Sweets

Sugar and sweets are abundant in modern diets, frequently appealing but possibly hazardous, especially during certain stages like menstruation. Common sources include sugary snacks, desserts, sweetened beverages, and even hidden sugars in processed meals. These things add to overall sugar intake and can influence health in many ways.

What Are They and the Best Foods to Get Rid of Them

Sugar is a simple carbohydrate found naturally in meals including fruits, vegetables, and dairy. However, the problematic sugars are added sugars—those added to meals during manufacturing or preparation. These include cane sugar, high-fructose corn syrup, and different syrups used to sweeten items.

To limit sugar intake, focus on nutritious meals such as fresh fruits and vegetables, lean meats, whole grains, and healthy fats. These meals give critical nutrition without extra added sugars.

Why Sugar Is a Problem

Excessive sugar intake can contribute to numerous health issues:

Dental Health: Sugar promotes tooth damage and cavities by feeding dangerous germs in the mouth.

Weight Gain: Sugary meals and beverages are abundant in calories but poor in nutritious value, resulting in weight gain and obesity.

Type 2 Diabetes: Overconsumption of sugar can lead to insulin resistance and raise the risk of rising type 2 diabetes.

Heart Health: High sugar intake is associated with an increased risk of heart disease, including hypertension and raised triglyceride levels.

Liver Health: The liver metabolizes sugar, and excessive ingestion can lead to fatty liver disease and other liver-related disorders.

Impact on Mood and Energy Levels

Sugar impacts mood and energy levels in numerous ways:

Blood Sugar Rises and Crashes: Consuming sugary meals produces quick rises in blood sugar levels, followed by a drop. This cycle can lead to weariness, irritation, and difficulty concentrating.

Serotonin and Dopamine Levels: Sugar causes the release of dopamine, a neurotransmitter linked with pleasure. However, repeated intake might desensitize dopamine receptors, resulting in cravings and mood swings.

Stress Response: Sugar intake can dysregulate cortisol, the stress hormone, aggravating stress, and anxiety levels.

Sugar and Inflammation

Sugar intake is intimately connected to inflammation, a crucial element in numerous chronic diseases:

Inflammatory Response: High sugar consumption induces the synthesis of inflammatory cytokines in the body, contributing to chronic inflammation.

Joint Pain: Inflammation induced by sugar can aggravate disorders like arthritis, leading to greater joint pain and stiffness.

Immune Function: Chronic inflammation weakens the immune system, leaving the body more prone to infections and disorders.

Skin Health: Sugar intake can aggravate skin disorders like acne and hasten skin aging owing to increased inflammation and glycation processes.

Practical Tips for Reducing Sugar Intake

Read Labels: Be careful of hidden sugars in processed foods, such as sauces, condiments, and packaged snacks.

Choose entire Foods: Opt for entire fruits instead of sugary snacks and sweets. Fresh veggies, lean meats, and nutritious grains should form the core of meals.

Limit Sweetened Beverages: Replace sugary sodas and energy drinks with water, herbal teas, or naturally flavored water.

Practice Moderation: Enjoy sweets infrequently and in moderate quantities. Savoring sweets attentively can lessen cravings and encourage healthy eating habits.

Cook at Home: Prepare meals at home using fresh ingredients to manage sugar levels and overall nutritional quality.

Knowing the influence of sugar on health, including its impacts on mood, energy levels, inflammation, and general well-being, is vital for making educated dietary decisions. By lowering the intake of sugary foods and choosing nutrient-dense alternatives, individuals may maintain their health and avoid the hazards associated with excessive sugar consumption. Embracing a balanced diet rich in natural foods and being cautious of added sugars can contribute to long-term health advantages, encouraging vigor and well-being throughout life. Taking proactive actions to limit sugar intake allows individuals to maximize their health and have a better quality of life.

Processed Meats and Dairy

Processed meats and dairy products are widespread in many diets but can have harmful impacts on health, especially during menstruation. Processed meats like sausages, bacon, and deli meats can include high quantities of salt, preservatives, and harmful fats. These substances can lead to inflammation and aggravate symptoms such as bloating and cramps during periods.

Similarly, processed dairy products like sweetened yogurts, flavored milk, and some cheeses may include additional sugars and artificial chemicals. These can disturb hormonal balance and worsen menstruation pain. Opting for fresh, unprocessed meats and dairy products or plant-based alternatives can help decrease these harmful effects and enhance overall menstrual health.

Refined Sugars and Carbohydrates

Refined sugars and carbs, frequently found in baked products, sugary snacks, and white bread, can elevate blood sugar levels fast. This quick spike is followed by a sudden decline, leading to weariness, mood fluctuations, and increased cravings. During menstruation, these variations might increase symptoms such as irritation and exhaustion.

Moreover, processed sugars cause inflammation in the body, which can worsen period cramps and bloating. Choosing whole grains like brown rice, quinoa, and whole wheat bread over processed carbohydrates will give prolonged energy and promote stable blood sugar levels. Opting for natural sweeteners like honey or maple syrup in moderation can also help lessen the harmful influence on menstrual health.

Fried Foods and Processed Snacks

Fried meals and processed snacks are generally heavy in harmful fats, salt, and artificial chemicals. These meals can lead to inflammation and intestinal discomfort, which may exacerbate during menstruation. Fried foods like French fries, fried chicken, and potato chips are also calorie-dense and lacking in nutrients, which can lead to weight gain and hormonal imbalance over time.

Processed foods such as packaged cookies, chips, and candy bars generally include processed sugars, harmful fats, and additives that give little nutritional benefit. These foods might worsen appetites and mood changes during menstruation. Opting for healthier options like air-popped popcorn, whole-grain crackers with nut butter, or homemade trail mix can satisfy cravings while delivering critical nutrients and improving overall well-being.

Exactly What to Eat at Every Stage of Your Menstrual Cycle

Menstrual Phase: During menstruation, focus on meals that boost replenishment and relieve symptoms. Opt for iron-rich meals like leafy greens, lean meats, and legumes to restore lost iron. Hydration is vital, so drink plenty of water and herbal teas to remain hydrated and to ease bloating.

Follicular Phase: As estrogen levels rise, promote hormone balance with nutrient-dense meals. Include nutritious grains like oats and quinoa, fresh fruits and vegetables, and lean meats. These nutrients give prolonged energy and enhance general well-being while the body prepares for ovulation.

Ovulatory Phase: During ovulation, focus on meals high in antioxidants and omega-3 fatty acids to support egg health and hormone balance. Include fatty seafood like salmon, nuts, and seeds, and antioxidant-rich berries. These foods can help decrease inflammation and improve reproductive health.

Luteal Phase: As progesterone levels grow, focus on foods that promote hormone balance and lessen PMS symptoms. Incorporate complex carbs like sweet potatoes and whole grains to balance blood sugar levels. Consist of magnesium-rich foods like dark chocolate and leafy greens to help reduce cramps and mood swings.

Foods That Help Reduce Period Cramps and What to Avoid Foods to Help Reduce Period Cramps:

1. Magnesium-rich foods: Dark leafy greens, nuts, seeds, and legumes can help relax muscles and prevent cramping.

2. Omega-3 Fatty Acids: Fatty fish like salmon, flaxseeds, and chia seeds contain anti-inflammatory characteristics that help decrease pain and inflammation.

3. Calcium: Dairy products, tofu, and fortified plant-based milk can help alleviate muscular tension and cramps.

4. Ginger: Known for its anti-inflammatory effects, ginger can help ease nausea and lessen menstruation discomfort.

Foods to Avoid:

1. High-Sodium Foods: Processed meats, canned soups, and salty snacks can lead to water retention and bloating.

2. Refined Sugars: Avoid sugary foods and beverages that might increase blood sugar changes and mood swings.

3. Trans Fats: Fried meals and commercially baked items commonly include trans fats that can cause inflammation and aggravate cramping.

4. Caffeine: Limit caffeine intake, since it might constrict blood vessels and raise stress, thereby exacerbating cramping.

Healthier Alternatives

Choosing healthier alternatives to popular dietary choices may greatly improve overall health and well-being, particularly during menstruation when controlling symptoms and maintaining energy levels are vital. Here are some helpful substitutions:

1. Whole Grains Instead of Refined Grains: Opt for whole grains like brown rice, quinoa, oats, and whole wheat bread instead of refined grains. Whole grains are rich in fiber, vitamins, and minerals, giving sustained energy and supporting digestive health.

2. Lean Proteins Instead of Processed Meats: Choose lean proteins such as chicken, turkey, tofu, lentils, and fish over processed meats like sausages and bacon. Lean proteins supply critical amino acids for muscle function and hormone synthesis without the extra salt and bad fats found in processed meats.

3. Healthy Fats Instead of Trans Fats: Include sources of healthy fats such as avocados, nuts, seeds, and olive oil in your diet. These fats improve brain function, hormone balance, and cardiovascular health compared to trans fats present in fried meals and commercially baked pastries.

4. Fresh Fruits and veggies Instead of Sugary Snacks: Snack on fresh fruits and veggies like carrots, celery, apples, and berries instead of sugary snacks and desserts. Fruits and vegetables are rich in vitamins, minerals, and antioxidants, improving general health and lowering cravings for refined sweets.

5. Herbal Teas and Water Instead of Sugary Beverages: Stay hydrated with herbal teas, water with lemon or cucumber slices, or unsweetened beverages instead of sugary sodas and energy drinks. Hydration maintains digestive health, decreases bloating, and helps maintain energy levels throughout the day.

Natural Sweeteners

Natural sweeteners give a healthier alternative to refined sugars, giving sweetness without the detrimental effects on blood sugar levels and general health. Here are some common natural sweeteners:

1. Honey: Honey is a natural sweetener rich in antioxidants and enzymes. It has a lower glycemic index compared to table sugar, meaning it promotes a slower rise in blood sugar levels. Use honey in moderation in tea, yogurt, or baking dishes for extra sweetness.

2. Maple Syrup: Maple syrup is created from the sap of maple trees and includes important antioxidants and minerals like zinc and manganese. It has a lower glycemic index than refined sugars and may be used as a topping for pancakes, porridge, or in baking.

3. Stevia: Stevia is a plant-based sweetener obtained from the leaves of the Stevia rebaudiana plant. It has zero calories and does not affect blood sugar levels, making it acceptable for persons with diabetes or those trying to minimize sugar intake. Use stevia in drinks, sweets, or to sweeten sauces and dressings.

4. Dates: Dates are naturally sweet fruits rich in fiber, potassium, and antioxidants. They have a lower glycemic index compared to processed sugars and may be mixed into smoothies, used to sweeten energy bars, or eaten as a natural snack.

5. Coconut Sugar: Coconut sugar is generated from the sap of coconut palm plants and includes minerals including iron, zinc, and calcium. It has a lower glycemic index than table sugar and may be used as a one-to-one substitution in baking and cooking.

Low-Glycemic Index Foods

Low-glycemic index (GI) meals are absorbed more slowly, creating a steady rise in blood sugar levels and delivering prolonged energy. These meals can help balance mood and energy levels during the menstrual period. Here are some examples of low-GI foods:

1. Legumes: Beans, lentils, and chickpeas are rich in fiber, protein, and complex carbs, boosting satiety and constant blood sugar levels.

2. Non-Starchy Vegetables: Leafy greens, broccoli, cauliflower, and bell peppers are low in carbs and calories but abundant in vitamins, minerals, and fiber.

3. Whole Fruits: Apples, oranges, berries, and pears have natural sugars but also give fiber, antioxidants, and important minerals.

4. Nuts and Seeds: Almonds, walnuts, chia seeds, and flaxseeds are rich in healthy fats, protein, and fiber, supporting heart health and balancing blood sugar levels.

5. Whole Grains: Quinoa, oats, barley, and whole wheat products are rich in fiber and minerals, giving sustained energy and aiding digestive health.

Including these low-GI items into meals and snacks can help control blood sugar levels, minimize cravings for sugary foods, and improve general health and well-being throughout the menstrual cycle.

Making informed dietary choices, such as selecting healthier options, adding natural sweeteners, and choosing low-GI meals, plays a key part in regulating menstrual health and general well-being. By choosing nutrient-dense foods that support hormone balance, energy levels, and digestive health, individuals may modify their diet to decrease symptoms related to menstruation and achieve long-term health benefits. Embracing a balanced approach to nutrition helps individuals take control of their eating habits and promote excellent menstrual health throughout life.

Chapter 4

Caffeine and Its Effects

A natural stimulant, caffeine may be found in a variety of beverages, together with coffee, tea, chocolate, and a variety of energy drinks. As a result of its capacity to enhance alertness and combat weariness, it is ingested by a large number of people all over the world. The effects of caffeine on the body, on the other hand, are multidimensional and can vary greatly depending on the extent of an individual's tolerance and how they consume caffeine. It is essential to have a solid understanding of these consequences, particularly for those who are managing their menstrual health.

In adding to its stimulant properties, caffeine can inhibit the neurotransmitter adenosine, which is responsible for the relaxation and drowsiness that it induces in the central nervous system. The inhibition of adenosine by coffee leads to an increase in the release of other neurotransmitters, such as dopamine and norepinephrine, which in turn leads to an increase in alertness and a reduction in weariness. As a result of this stimulant impact, a lot of individuals rely on their morning coffee to get their day started, or they go for an energy drink when they are feeling down in the middle of the day.

This means that caffeine has diuretic effects, which means that it causes an increase in the amount of urine that is produced. Excessive consumption can contribute to fluid loss and possible dehydration, particularly if it is not balanced with proper water intake. Moderate consumption, on the other hand, does not often result in substantial dehydration.

The effects of caffeine may be broken down into two categories: short-term and long-term. Caffeine had shown to boost cognitive function, mood, and physical performance in the short term. However, long-term excessive usage can lead to dependence, with withdrawal symptoms such as headaches, irritability, and exhaustion upon discontinuation. Additionally, large dosages of caffeine might result in undesirable consequences including sleeplessness, jitteriness, and elevated heart rate.

Caffeine and Menstrual Cramps

Menstrual cramps, or dysmenorrhea, are a typical condition experienced by many people during their menstrual cycle. The association between coffee consumption and menstrual cramps is complicated and might vary across people.

Prostaglandins and Pain: During menstruation, the body releases prostaglandins, hormone-like chemicals that stimulate the uterine muscles to spasm, resulting in cramps. Caffeine can constrict blood vessels and elevate blood pressure, thereby exacerbating the discomfort associated with these contractions.

Inflammation: Caffeine can increase inflammation in the body, which can increase menstrual cramps. By boosting the production of certain stress hormones, coffee might raise the body's inflammatory response, thereby making cramps more severe and harder to control.

Magnesium Depletion: Caffeine can interfere with the absorption of magnesium, a vital mineral that helps relax muscles and prevent cramping. Lower magnesium levels might contribute to more severe period cramps and discomfort.

Individual Sensitivity: The influence of coffee on menstrual cramps might vary substantially. Some individuals may find that limiting coffee intake alleviates cramp intensity, while others may not detect a substantial change. Monitoring personal responses to coffee can help identify whether it adds to menstruation pain.

How Caffeine Affects the Body

Caffeine's effects on the body are vast, involving different physiological systems and functions.

Central Nervous System: As a central nervous system stimulant, caffeine enhances alertness, lowers the impression of exhaustion, and can boost attention and cognitive performance. It does this by inhibiting adenosine receptors and enhancing the release of neurotransmitters like dopamine and norepinephrine.

Cardiovascular System: Caffeine can produce a brief rise in heart rate and blood pressure. For most healthy people, moderate caffeine use is not detrimental. However, people with cardiovascular problems or hypertension may need to watch their consumption attentively.

Digestive System: Caffeine boosts the formation of stomach acid, which can lead to digestive pain or worsen illnesses like acid reflux and gastritis. It also speeds up the movement of food through the digestive tract, which can occasionally contribute to diarrhea.

Metabolism and Energy: Caffeine can temporarily enhance metabolism and promote fat oxidation, making it a popular element in weight reduction pills. This metabolic action can lead to a modest increase in calorie burning, however, its long-term influence on weight control is limited.

Sleep Patterns: Caffeine's stimulant effects can interfere with sleep, mostly if eaten in high amounts or later in the day. It can affect the quality and amount of sleep, resulting in difficulties including insomnia and daytime drowsiness.

Caffeine's Impact on Anxiety and Stress

While coffee is recognized for its potential to improve alertness and energy levels, it may also have a substantial influence on anxiety and stress.

Anxiety Levels: Caffeine boosts the production of adrenaline, the "fight-or-flight" hormone. While this might enhance energy and attention, it can also contribute to heightened anxiety, uneasiness, and jitteriness in certain individuals. Those who are prone to anxiety problems may discover that coffee exacerbates their symptoms.

Stress Response: Caffeine promotes the production of cortisol, a stress hormone. Elevated cortisol levels over longer durations can contribute to chronic stress and related health concerns. High cortisol levels can also influence menstrual health by altering the hormonal balance, perhaps leading to irregular periods and worsening PMS symptoms.

Mental Health: For those with anxiety disorders or panic disorders, coffee can cause or aggravate symptoms, including panic attacks. Reducing or eliminating caffeine intake can be good for controlling anxiety and generating a calmer state of mind.

Tolerance and Sensitivity: Individual tolerance to caffeine varies significantly. Some people may consume enormous quantities without substantial worry or tension, while others may have heightened anxiety with even small doses of coffee. Understanding personal sensitivity and regulating consumption properly might help mitigate these effects.

Integrating Knowledge for Better Health

Understanding the various effects of caffeine on the body, particularly during menstruation, is vital for making informed dietary decisions. While caffeine delivers advantages including enhanced alertness and improved cognitive performance, its propensity to worsen menstrual cramps, contribute to inflammation, and alter anxiety and stress levels needs cautious evaluation.

By monitoring individualized reactions to caffeine, individuals may better control their consumption to reduce negative effects and improve general well-being. Exploring healthier alternatives, such as herbal teas or decaffeinated products, can deliver the necessary advantages without the harmful effects on menstrual health and mental well-being.

Balancing caffeine use with an understanding of its effects on the body, especially during menstruation, allows individuals to make choices that promote their health and comfort.

Reducing Caffeine Intake

Reducing caffeine intake can considerably assist people suffering unfavorable consequences from high caffeine usage, particularly during menstruation. High caffeine levels can intensify period cramps, raise anxiety, and disturb sleep habits. Transitioning to a reduced caffeine diet entails knowing its availability in various foods and beverages, identifying withdrawal symptoms, and adopting ways to decrease intake successfully.

Understanding Caffeine Sources: The first step in lowering caffeine intake is recognizing its key sources. While coffee and tea are well-known caffeine sources, other liquids and foods also contribute to daily consumption. Energy drinks, sodas, chocolate, and some pharmaceuticals can contain substantial levels of caffeine. Reading labels and being aware of hidden sources is key for properly regulating consumption.

Recognizing Withdrawal Symptoms: Reducing coffee intake can lead to withdrawal symptoms, including headaches, irritability, exhaustion, and problems focusing. These symptoms are transitory and often diminish within a few days to a week. Gradually lowering caffeine consumption can help decrease the intensity of withdrawal symptoms, making the transition gentler.

Tips for Cutting Down

Cutting down on caffeine demands a systematic strategy to guarantee a seamless transition and reduce withdrawal symptoms. Here are some practical strategies to help minimize caffeine intake:

1. Gradual Reduction: Abruptly quitting caffeine might lead to significant withdrawal symptoms. Instead, gradually lessen your dose over many weeks. For example, if you regularly drink four cups of coffee a day, start by reducing down to three cups for a week, then two, and so on.

2. Switch to Decaffeinated Options: Replace caffeinated beverages with their decaffeinated counterparts. Decaffeinated coffee and tea give the same familiar habits without the excessive caffeine content. This can help lower total intake while still enjoying the flavors and rituals connected with these drinks.

3. Mix Caffeinated and Decaffeinated: If you find it tough to give up your favorite caffeinated beverage totally, consider combining caffeinated and decaffeinated varieties. Gradually increase the percentage of decaffeinated to caffeinated until you are predominantly consuming decaffeinated liquids.

4. lower Serving Sizes: Another helpful method is to lower the serving size of caffeinated beverages. Opt for a smaller cup of coffee or tea, or dilute your beverage with water or milk. This allows you to enjoy your drink with less caffeine.

5. Avoid Caffeine in the Afternoon: Caffeine ingested later in the day might disturb sleep patterns. Set a cut-off time for caffeine use, ideally by early afternoon, to ensure it doesn't interfere with your ability to fall asleep and obtain restorative sleep.

6. Find Alternative Sources of Energy: If you rely on coffee for an energy boost, try alternate ways to enhance your energy levels organically. Regular exercise, proper sleep, a balanced diet, and stress management strategies can all contribute to greater energy without the need for coffee.

Caffeine-Free Alternatives

Transitioning to caffeine-free options can provide equal advantages and enjoyment without the detrimental consequences linked with caffeine. Here are some healthful and delicious caffeine-free options:

1. Herbal Teas: Herbal teas are terrific caffeine-free alternative to standard tea and coffee. Options, including chamomile, peppermint, ginger, and rooibos, offer a range of tastes and health advantages. Chamomile can induce relaxation and improve sleep, while peppermint assists digestion and lowers headaches.

2. Water Infusions: Infusing water with fruits, vegetables, and herbs may make pleasant and tasty beverages without caffeine. Combinations like cucumber and mint, lemon and ginger, or berries and basil lend a pleasant flavor to simple water and support improved hydration.

3. Golden Milk: Golden milk is a warm, calming beverage made with turmeric, milk (or a plant-based replacement), and spices like cinnamon and ginger.

Turmeric contains anti-inflammatory effects and can aid with period cramps and general wellness.

4. Coconut Water: Coconut water is a natural, hydrating beverage rich in electrolytes like potassium and magnesium. It is an excellent alternative to caffeinated sports drinks and can help replace lost fluids and minerals.

5. Green Smoothies: Green smoothies prepared with leafy greens, fruits, and a liquid base (such as water or almond milk) give a healthful and energy-boosting alternative to coffee. Ingredients like spinach, kale, bananas, and berries make a delightful and nutrient-packed drink.

6. Decaffeinated Coffee and Tea: For individuals who appreciate the flavor of coffee or tea but wish to avoid caffeine, decaffeinated versions are a wonderful alternative. They deliver the classic flavors without the stimulating impacts.

7. Warm Lemon Water: Starting the day with warm lemon water may be a delightful and caffeine-free method to enhance hydration and jumpstart digestion. Lemon water delivers vitamin C and antioxidants, increasing general wellness.

8. Apple Cider Vinegar Drink: Mixing a tablespoon of apple cider vinegar with water and a touch of honey may produce a tart, refreshing drink that helps with digestion and energy levels.

9. Vegetable Juices: Fresh vegetable juices produced from components like carrots, beets, celery, and cucumbers are filled with vitamins, minerals, and antioxidants. They offer a healthful and hydrated alternative to caffeinated beverages.

10. Bone Broth: Bone broth is nutrient-dense fluid rich in collagen, amino acids, and minerals. It may be drunk on its own or used as a foundation for soups and stews, giving hydration and sustenance

Creating a Sustainable Caffeine Reduction Plan

Successfully lowering caffeine usage and switching to healthy alternatives includes building a sustainable plan that corresponds with individual preferences and lifestyles. Here are some procedures to guarantee a seamless and effective transition:

1. Create clear targets: Define your motivations for limiting caffeine use and create clear, realistic targets. Whether it's increasing menstrual health, lowering anxiety, or enhancing sleep quality, having a clear aim helps encourage and direct your efforts.

2. Monitor Progress: Keep track of your coffee usage and record any changes in your symptoms or overall well-being. Monitoring progress might help you understand what works best for you and make necessary modifications.

3. Seek Support: Share your objectives with friends, family, or a support group. Having a support system may give encouragement, accountability, and useful advice for lowering caffeine usage.

4. Be Patient: Reducing caffeine intake is a gradual process, and it's crucial to be patient with yourself. Withdrawal symptoms may occur, but they are transitory and will lessen as your body adjusts.

5. Enjoy the Journey: Explore and enjoy the diversity of caffeine-free choices available. Experimenting with various flavors and beverages can make the transition fun and help you find new favorites.

6. Maintain Balance: Balance is vital to any dietary modification. While lowering caffeine, ensuring your diet is rich in other nutrients, and promoting general health. Incorporate a variety of healthful meals, remain hydrated, and pursue a healthy lifestyle.

Reducing caffeine intake and adding caffeine-free alternatives can lead to improved health, particularly for persons managing menstruation symptoms, anxiety, or sleep difficulties. By understanding the effects of caffeine and using practical measures, you may build a balanced and healthy approach to caffeine usage, boosting general well-being and quality of life.

Chapter 5

Processed Foods and Preservatives

Processed foods have become an important element of the contemporary diet, typically praised for their convenience and lengthy shelf life. These foods undergo different techniques of preparation and preservation to increase flavor, extend usage, and minimize preparation time. However, the thorough processing typically entails adding preservatives, artificial flavors, and other compounds that might have detrimental impacts on health.

The Hidden Dangers

The hidden risks of processed meals are often camouflaged by their convenience and pleasure. While they might save time and effort, the long-term health repercussions can be significant. Consuming a diet heavy in processed foods has been related to several health risks, including obesity, heart disease, diabetes, and some malignancies.

Heavy levels of Sugar, Salt, and Fats: Processed foods are often heavy in added sugars, salt, and harmful fats. These components can contribute to weight gain, high blood pressure, and raised cholesterol levels. Excessive sugar intake is particularly harmful as it can lead to insulin resistance, a precursor to type 2 diabetes.

Nutrient Deficiency: Many processed foods are deprived of critical nutrients during manufacture. The refining process eliminates fiber, vitamins, and minerals, resulting in "empty calories" that offer energy but lack the required components for maintaining health.

Artificial Additives: Processed foods typically contain artificial additives, including colors, tastes, and preservatives. While these additions assist enhance taste, appearance, and shelf life, they can have various health effects. Some chemicals are associated with allergic responses, while others may have more harmful long-term impacts.

Additives and Their Effects on Health

Food additives are compounds added to food to retain flavor, increase taste, and improve appearance. While some chemicals are innocuous or even useful, some can offer health hazards, especially when ingested in significant quantities over time.

Artificial Sweeteners: Used as a replacement for sugar, artificial sweeteners like aspartame and sucralose are widespread in diet beverages and low-calorie meals. Though usually regarded safe in modest dosages, certain studies show they may interfere with metabolism and insulin sensitivity, potentially leading to weight gain and increased risk of diabetes.

Monosodium Glutamate (MSG): MSG is a flavor enhancer typically found in savory snacks, canned soups, and restaurant cuisine. While MSG is widely accepted as harmless, some individuals experience symptoms including headaches, perspiration, and nausea after ingestion, a condition known as the "Chinese Restaurant Syndrome."

Trans Fats: These fats are intentionally generated by hydrogenation and are present in many baked products, margarine, and fried meals. Trans fats are known for raising bad cholesterol levels (LDL) while reducing good cholesterol levels (HDL), dramatically increasing the risk of heart disease.

Preservatives: Common preservatives include nitrates and nitrites in processed meats, sulfites in dry fruits, and benzoates in acidic foods. While these compounds reduce spoilage and bacterial development, they have been related to different health concerns. For instance, nitrates and nitrites can produce carcinogenic chemicals called nitrosamines under certain circumstances.

Processed Foods and Hormonal Imbalance

The use of processed foods can drastically disrupt hormonal balance, which is vital for sustaining general health, particularly in women. Hormones govern several biological activities, including metabolism, reproductive health, and mood. Disruption in hormone levels can lead to several health concerns, including menstruation abnormalities, infertility, and mental disorders.

Endocrine Disruptors: Many processed foods include endocrine-disrupting chemicals (EDCs) that can interfere with hormone function. These chemicals, such as bisphenol A (BPA) and phthalates, are typically present in food packaging and can leak into the food. EDCs imitate or block hormones and disturb the body's natural activities, resulting in concerns including irregular menstrual cycles, polycystic ovarian syndrome (PCOS), and a higher risk of hormone-related malignancies.

Impact on Insulin and Blood Sugar: Processed meals heavy in refined sugars and carbs can produce fast rises in blood sugar levels, leading the pancreas to release significant quantities of insulin. Over time, this can lead to insulin resistance and disturb other hormones, including estrogen and progesterone, which are crucial for reproductive health.

Inflammation: Many processed meals are heavy in inflammatory components, such as refined carbohydrates, bad fats, and artificial chemicals. Chronic inflammation can affect the balance of hormones like cortisol, the stress hormone, which can have a cascade effect on other hormonal activities, including those associated with reproduction and mood control.

Choosing Whole Foods

Shifting from a diet high in processed foods to one rich in whole foods can greatly enhance general health and well-being. Whole foods are little processed and near to their natural condition. They are often free from added sugars, bad fats, and artificial additives, making them a better choice.

Benefits of Whole Foods: Whole foods give a plethora of nutrients important for preserving health. They are rich in vitamins, minerals, antioxidants, and fiber, which support numerous biological processes, from strengthening the immune system to preserving digestive health.

Fruits and Vegetables: Fresh fruits and vegetables are cornerstone components of a whole-food diet. They are low in calories yet abundant in important nutrients. Leafy greens, berries, citrus fruits, and cruciferous vegetables like broccoli and cauliflower are particularly useful for their high vitamin and antioxidant content.

Whole Grains: Whole grains, such as brown rice, quinoa, oats, and whole wheat, are high in fiber, which aids in digestion and helps manage blood sugar levels. Unlike processed grains, whole grains maintain their bran and germ, giving more nutrients and increasing satiety.

Lean Proteins: Including lean proteins such as chicken, fish, beans, and lentils is vital for muscle repair and development, hormone synthesis, and overall energy levels. These proteins are lower in harmful fats compared to processed meats and contain vital amino acids.

Healthy Fats: Healthy fats, such as those found in avocados, nuts, seeds, and olive oil, are vital for brain function, hormone synthesis, and lowering inflammation. Unlike trans fats and hydrogenated oils found in processed meals, these fats boost heart health and general wellness.

Dairy Alternatives: For individuals sensitive to dairy or wishing to avoid the additives in processed dairy products, there are numerous nutritious alternatives available. Plant-based milk, such as almond, soy, and oat milk, as well as dairy-free yogurts and cheeses, can give similar nutritional advantages without the harmful effects of conventional dairy products.

Implementing Whole Foods into Your Diet

Transitioning to a diet rich in whole foods may be a pleasurable and sustainable way to improve health. Here are some practical methods to include more whole foods into your everyday routine:

Plan and Prepare: Planning meals and snacks ahead of time will assist ensure that you have healthy alternatives readily available. Preparing meals in advance can lessen dependency on convenience foods and make it simpler to keep to a whole-food diet.

Shop the Perimeter: Grocery shops often arrange entire foods like fruits, vegetables, meats, and dairy along the perimeter of the store. Focusing your shopping in these regions will help you avoid the processed meals commonly found in the central aisles.

Stay Informed: Educating yourself about nutrition and the advantages of whole foods will empower you to make healthier choices. Resources like nutrition books, reliable websites, and meetings with dietitians can give vital knowledge and assistance.

Benefits of a Whole Food Diet

A whole food diet emphasizes natural, minimally processed foods, delivering several health advantages that can contribute to enhanced overall well-being. Here are some of the major advantages of following a whole-food diet:

Improved Nutrient Intake

Whole foods are rich in critical elements, including vitamins, minerals, fiber, and antioxidants. Unlike processed foods, which typically lose vital nutrients during production, whole foods preserve their nutritional integrity. Consuming a mix of fruits, vegetables, whole grains, lean proteins, and healthy fats ensures that your body obtains a balanced amount of nutrients essential for optimal functioning.

Enhanced Digestive Health

The high fiber level in whole meals supports healthy digestion and regular bowel movements. Fiber provides weight to the stool and helps it flow through the digestive tract more readily, minimizing the risk of constipation. Moreover, a diet rich in fiber stimulates the growth of good gut bacteria, which play a critical role in maintaining healthy gut microbiota and overall digestive health.

Better Weight Management

Whole foods are often fewer in calories and greater in satiety compared to processed foods, making them suitable for weight management. Food's high in fiber and protein help you feel full longer, lowering the likelihood of overeating and snacking between meals. By concentrating on nutrient-dense whole foods, you may naturally regulate your calorie consumption without feeling deprived.

Reduced Risk of Chronic Diseases

A whole food diet is connected with a decreased risk of chronic illnesses such as heart disease, diabetes, and some malignancies. The antioxidants and anti-inflammatory substances found in fruits, vegetables, nuts, and seeds help protect the body against oxidative stress and inflammation, which are the underlying causes of many chronic disorders. Additionally, the absence of toxic trans fats, processed carbohydrates, and excessive salt in whole meals helps to better cardiovascular health and stable blood sugar levels.

Enhanced Energy Levels

Whole foods give a constant flow of energy, helping to maintain regular blood sugar levels throughout the day. Unlike the fast energy spikes and crashes associated with sugary and processed diets, whole foods deliver lasting energy, keeping you awake and focused. Incorporating a range of whole grains, lean proteins, and healthy fats into your meals delivers a balanced source of energy.

Improved Mental Health

Emerging evidence shows that a whole-food diet might significantly benefit mental health. Nutrient-rich diets, particularly those strong in omega-3 fatty acids, vitamins, and minerals, improve brain health and cognitive performance. A diet heavy in fruits, vegetables, and whole grains has been associated with a decreased incidence of sadness and anxiety. The lack of artificial chemicals and excessive sweets also leads to better mood control and general mental well-being.

Easy Swaps for Processed Foods

Transitioning to a whole-food diet doesn't have to be daunting. Making little, attainable adjustments can have a major influence on your health. Here are some easy substitutions to replace processed meals with healthier whole-food alternatives:

Breakfast

Swap Sugary Cereals for Oatmeal: Sugary cereals are generally filled with processed sugars and artificial flavors. Instead, go for oatmeal prepared with whole oats. You may sweeten it naturally with fresh fruits, a drop of honey, or a sprinkle of cinnamon. Adding nuts and seeds can advance the nutritional content and keep you satisfied longer.

Replace White Toast with Whole Grain Bread: White bread is created from refined flour, which lacks the benefits found in whole grains. Choose whole-grain bread, which provides more fiber, vitamins, and minerals. Look for kinds with less added sugars and preservatives.

Snacks

Choose Fresh Fruit Over Candy: When desiring something sweet, seek for fresh fruit instead of candy or sugary treats. Fruits like apples, berries, and oranges are naturally sweet and rich in vitamins, antioxidants, and fiber. They fulfill your sweet taste while giving critical nutrients.

Swap Chips for Nuts & Seeds: Potato chips and other processed foods are heavy in harmful fats, salt, and artificial additives. Nuts and seeds, such as almonds, walnuts, and sunflower seeds, are wonderful choices. They deliver healthy fats, protein, and fiber, keeping you satiated between meals.

Lunch and Dinner

Opt for Grilled Chicken Instead of Processed Deli Meats: Processed deli meats generally include preservatives, high levels of salt, and harmful fats. Grilled chicken breast is a lean protein source free from additives. Season it with herbs and spices for added taste.

Replace White Rice with Quinoa or Brown Rice: White rice is a refined grain with fewer nutrients than its whole grain competitors. Quinoa and brown rice are higher in fiber, vitamins, and minerals. They also have a lower glycemic index, delivering more steady energy levels.

Substitute Processed Sauces with Homemade Versions: Many store-bought sauces and dressings have extra sugars, bad fats, and preservatives. Making your sauces at home allows you to control the ingredients. Simple mixes of olive oil, vinegar, herbs, and spices may produce tasty and healthful dressings.

Beverages

Choose Water or Herbal Tea Over Soda: Sugary drinks are heavy in calories and offer little nutritional value. Drinking water or herbal tea keeps you hydrated without the additional sweets and artificial additives. For a refreshing twist, infuse water with slices of lemon, cucumber, or mint.

Replace Fruit Juices with entire Fruits: Fruit juices, particularly those branded as "natural," typically include additional sugars and lack the fiber found in entire fruits. Eating entire fruits delivers the whole nutritional advantages, including fiber, which helps manage blood sugar levels.

Desserts

Opt for Dark Chocolate Instead of Milk Chocolate: Dark chocolate with a high cocoa content is lower in sugar and includes more antioxidants compared to milk chocolate. It can fulfill chocolate cravings while delivering some health advantages. Look for variants with at least 70% cocoa.

Choose Greek Yogurt with Fresh Fruit Over Ice Cream: Ice cream is often heavy in sweets and bad fats. Greek yogurt, especially the unsweetened version, provides a protein-rich option. Top it with fresh fruit and a sprinkling of almonds for a tasty and healthful dessert.

Cooking Methods

Bake or Grill Instead of Frying: Frying meals add unwanted fats and calories. Baking or grilling maintains the natural taste of food without the need for extra oil. These approaches are healthy and may make veggies, meats, and fish more delectable.

Use Herbs & Spices Instead of Salt: Excessive salt intake is related to high blood pressure and heart disease. Flavor your recipes with herbs and spices like basil, thyme, rosemary, and paprika. They offer richness and diversity to your dishes without the negative health implications of salt.

Foods that Support Hormone Balance and Mood

Maintaining hormone balance and a steady mood is vital for general well-being, especially for women throughout their menstrual cycles. Certain meals can have a major influence on hormone levels and emotional health, fostering a sense of balance and well-being. Incorporating select nutrient-rich foods into your diet can help balance hormones and boost mood. Here, we investigate the greatest foods to boost hormone balance and mood, including leafy greens, cruciferous vegetables, berries, antioxidant-rich fruits, and fermented foods containing probiotics.

Leafy Greens and Cruciferous Vegetables

Leafy greens and cruciferous vegetables are nutritional powerhouses that offer a range of health advantages, notably for hormone balance and mood stability. These veggies are rich in vitamins, minerals, and antioxidants that support the body's endocrine system and promote general health.

Spinach and Kale: Spinach and kale are good providers of magnesium, a mineral necessary for hormonal balance. Magnesium helps control cortisol levels, the stress hormone, and can alleviate feelings of anxiety and sadness. Additionally, these greens are strong in folate, which encourages the creation of serotonin, a neurotransmitter that boosts mood.

Broccoli and Brussels Sprouts: Cruciferous plants like broccoli and Brussels sprouts contain chemicals known as glucosinolates, which are transformed into active compounds like indole-3-carbinol (I3C) and diindolylmethane (DIM) during digestion. These molecules assist the liver to cleanse and remove excess hormones, particularly estrogen, supporting hormone balance.

Arugula and Swiss Chard: Arugula and Swiss chard are filled with vitamins A, C, and K, as well as iron and calcium. Vitamin C is needed for adrenal gland function, which controls the release of cortisol. Vitamin K supports good blood clotting and bone health, while iron and calcium are necessary for energy levels and muscular function.

Regular eating of leafy greens and cruciferous vegetables can help balance hormone levels, decrease inflammation, and enhance mood. These veggies are flexible and may be readily included in salads, smoothies, stir-fries, and soups.

Berries and Antioxidant-Rich Fruits

Berries and other antioxidant-rich fruits are not only tasty but also incredibly good for hormone balance and mood enhancement. These fruits are filled with vitamins, minerals, and antioxidants that protect the body from oxidative stress and promote hormonal balance.

Blueberries and Strawberries: Blueberries and strawberries are rich in antioxidants like anthocyanins, which help decrease inflammation and protect the body from free radical damage. These berries also include vitamin C, which promotes adrenal function and helps the body regulate stress. The natural sweetness of berries helps satisfy sugar cravings, helping to maintain stable blood sugar levels and minimize mood swings.

Raspberries and Blackberries: Raspberries and blackberries are strong in fiber, which aids in digestion and helps maintain a healthy gut microbiota. A healthy gut is vital for hormone control since it regulates the generation and metabolism of hormones. These berries also include vitamins E and K, which assist skin health and bone strength.

Cherries and Pomegranates: Cherries and pomegranates are rich in polyphenols, potent antioxidants that decrease inflammation and improve cardiovascular health. Cherries contain melatonin, a hormone that controls sleep-wake cycles, helping to enhance sleep quality and mood. Pomegranates have been demonstrated to have anti-estrogenic properties, which can help regulate estrogen levels in the body.

A variety of berries and antioxidant-rich fruits into your diet will help protect your body from oxidative stress, improve hormone balance, and increase mood. These fruits may be enjoyed fresh, frozen, or dried, and make fantastic complements to yogurt, porridge, smoothies, and desserts.

Fermented Foods and Probiotics

Fermented foods and probiotics serve a critical role in maintaining a healthy gut flora, which is directly connected to hormone balance and mood modulation. The gut-brain axis, a communication link between the stomach and the brain, underscores the relevance of gut health for general well-being.

Yogurt and Kefir: Yogurt and kefir are fermented dairy products rich in probiotics, helpful microorganisms that improve intestinal health. These probiotics assist in maintaining a healthy gut flora, which regulates the synthesis and metabolism of hormones. Regular use of yogurt and kefir can improve digestion, increase immunity, and enhance mood by boosting the synthesis of serotonin.

Sauerkraut and Kimchi: Sauerkraut and kimchi are fermented vegetables that contain high quantities of probiotics, vitamins, and minerals. These fermented foods stimulate the growth of good gut bacteria, assisting in digestion and nutritional absorption. The fermentation process also boosts the bioavailability of nutrients, making them simpler for the body to consume. Including sauerkraut and kimchi in your diet can boost gut health, reduce inflammation, and maintain hormone balance.

Miso and Tempeh: Miso and tempeh are fermented soy products that provide a rich source of probiotics and protein. Miso is prepared from fermented soybeans and barley or rice, whereas tempeh is created from fermented whole soybeans. These foods include isoflavones, plant components that mimic estrogen in the body and can help regulate hormone levels. Miso and tempeh also help intestinal health, ease digestion, and enhance mood.

By including fermented foods and probiotics in your diet, you can promote healthy gut flora, which plays a crucial role in hormone balance and mood improvement. These foods may be consumed in numerous forms, such as yogurt with fresh fruit, kimchi in stir-fries, sauerkraut as a side dish, and miso soup.

Foods that Combat Fatigue and Bloating

Fatigue and bloating are frequent symptoms that can greatly impair everyday living, especially for women during their menstrual periods. These symptoms can be addressed via attentive food choices. Incorporating iron-rich meals, vitamin B-rich foods, and potassium-rich foods into your diet will help battle fatigue and minimize bloating, leading to a more comfortable and energized lifestyle. Here, we investigate these critical nutrients and the foods that produce them, giving practical recommendations for integrating them into your meals.

Iron-rich foods (Red Meat, Beans, etc.)

Iron is an essential mineral that plays a significant function in sustaining energy levels and minimizing weariness. It is a crucial component of hemoglobin, the protein in red blood cells responsible for delivering oxygen throughout the body. Without appropriate iron, the body cannot create enough healthy red blood cells, resulting in iron deficiency anemia, characterized by tiredness, weakness, and pallor.

Red Meat: Red meat, such as beef and lamb, is a rich source of heme iron, the form of iron that is most readily absorbed by the body. Including lean portions of red meat in your diet will help improve iron levels and prevent weariness. For people who consume meat, consuming beef liver, which is particularly strong in iron, might be advantageous.

Chicken and Fish: While red meat is a well-known source of iron, chicken and fish both supply large amounts of this crucial element. Chicken and turkey, particularly dark flesh, contain heme iron. Fish such as salmon, tuna, and sardines not only supply iron but also contain omega-3 fatty acids, which have anti-inflammatory effects that can help relieve bloating.

Beans and Lentils: For people following a vegetarian or vegan diet, beans and lentils are great sources of non-heme iron. Although non-heme iron is not as easily absorbed by the body as heme iron, combining these plant-based sources with vitamin C-rich meals can boost absorption. For example, adding bell peppers, tomatoes, or citrus fruits to your meals will boost iron intake.

Spinach and Other Leafy Greens: Spinach, kale, and other leafy greens are high in non-heme iron and also contain several other nutrients that support general health. While the iron in these greens is not as quickly absorbed as heme iron, their high vitamin C concentration benefits in increasing absorption.

Vitamin B-rich foods (Whole Grains, Lean Meats, etc.)

Vitamin B complex covers a collection of critical vitamins that play a key function in energy generation and minimizing weariness. These vitamins help turn the food we consume into energy and promote the operation of the neurological system. Ensuring an appropriate diet of B vitamins can assist sustain energy levels and prevent symptoms of weariness.

Whole Grains: Whole grains such as brown rice, quinoa, oatmeal, and whole wheat products are good providers of B vitamins, including B1 (thiamine), B2 (riboflavin), B3 (niacin), B6 (pyridoxine), and B9 (folate). These vitamins are necessary for energy metabolism and the production of red blood cells. Incorporating a variety of whole grains into your diet might assist sustain energy levels throughout the day.

Lean Meats: Lean meats such as chicken, turkey, and lean cuts of cattle and hog provide a rich supply of B vitamins, notably B12, which is needed for red blood cell synthesis and brain function. Vitamin B12 is largely found in animal sources, thus people following a vegetarian or vegan diet may seek fortified foods or pills to satisfy their needs.

Eggs and Dairy Products: Eggs and dairy products, such as milk, cheese, and yogurt, are also rich sources of B vitamins. Eggs provide practically all the B vitamins, including B12, whereas dairy products supply B2 and B12. Including these items in your diet can assist promote energy generation and prevent weariness.

Potassium-rich foods (Bananas, Avocados, etc.)

Potassium is a vital element that helps maintain fluid balance, muscular contractions, and nerve messages. It has a key function in minimizing bloating by counteracting the effects of sodium and encouraging the removal of excess fluid from the body. Adequate potassium consumption can assist in maintaining optimum hydration and decrease bloating and tiredness.

Avocados: Avocados are rich in potassium and healthful monounsaturated fats, which improve heart health and give long-lasting energy. They also include fiber, which aids with digestion and helps avoid bloating. Adding avocado to salads, sandwiches, or smoothies is a simple way to enhance your potassium consumption.

Sweet Potatoes: Sweet potatoes are a fantastic source of potassium and also supply complex carbs, which assist sustain energy levels. It is rich in fiber, vitamins A and C, and antioxidants. Incorporating sweet potatoes into your meals might help battle tiredness and minimize bloating.

Oranges and Citrus Fruits: Oranges and other citrus fruits are not only high in potassium but also rich in vitamin C, which improves immunological function and enhances iron absorption. Drinking a glass of freshly squeezed orange juice or having a citrus fruit as a snack might help maintain potassium levels and decrease bloating.

Chapter 6

Fatty and Fried Foods

Fatty and fried meals have become a mainstay in many diets globally due to their ease and often enticing flavor. However, these foods can severely damage health, particularly when taken in excess. Understanding the ramifications of consuming unhealthy fats and fried foods is vital for making educated dietary choices that promote long-term well-being. This section addresses the impact of unhealthy fats, the function of saturated fats in inflammation, and the digestive concerns linked with fried meals.

The Impact of Unhealthy Fats

Unhealthy fats, particularly trans fats and excessive saturated fats, have been related to several health concerns, including heart disease, obesity, and diabetes. These fats are commonly found in processed meals, baked products, and fried items, contributing to an unhealthy diet when taken consistently.

Trans Fats: Trans fats are intentionally manufactured by hydrogenation, which transforms liquid oils into solid fats to increase the shelf life of food goods. They are often found in margarine, shortening, processed snacks, and baked items. Trans fats are particularly dangerous because they elevate LDL (bad) cholesterol levels while decreasing HDL (good) cholesterol levels, dramatically raising the risk of cardiovascular disease. Additionally, trans fats have been connected with inflammation, insulin resistance, and an increased risk of developing type 2 diabetes.

Saturated Fats: Saturated fats are normally solid at room temperature and are found in animal products such as meat, butter, cheese, and dairy, as well as some plant-based oils like coconut and palm oil. While limited amounts of saturated fats can be part of a balanced diet, excessive intake can lead to raised cholesterol levels and an increased risk of heart disease. Saturated fats can also contribute to the development of fatty liver disease and obesity when taken in big quantities.

Obesity and Metabolic Syndrome: The high-calorie density of greasy and fried meals might lead to weight gain and obesity. Obesity is a vital risk factor for metabolic syndrome, a cluster of disorders that raise the risk of heart disease, stroke, and diabetes. Metabolic syndrome comprises high blood pressure, excessive blood sugar, extra body fat around the waist, and abnormal cholesterol levels. Reducing the consumption of harmful fats can help control weight and minimize the risk of certain illnesses.

Saturated Fats and Inflammation

Inflammation is a normal reaction by the body to damage or infection, but persistent inflammation can lead to several health concerns, including cardiovascular disease, arthritis, and some malignancies. Diet has a crucial impact in either increasing or lowering inflammation, and saturated fats are known to contribute to chronic inflammation.

Pro-Inflammatory Effects: Saturated fats can generate an inflammatory response in the body by activating particular immune cells and pathways. These immune cells emit pro-inflammatory cytokines, which can cause harm to tissues and organs over time. High consumption of saturated fats has been associated with higher levels of these cytokines, contributing to chronic inflammation and related illnesses.

Endothelial Dysfunction: Saturated fats can damage the function of the endothelium, the thin layer of cells lining the blood arteries. Endothelial dysfunction is a critical element in the development of atherosclerosis, a disorder defined by the formation of fatty plaques in the arteries. This can lead to reducing of blood flow, elevated blood pressure, and a higher risk of heart attack and stroke.

Insulin Resistance: Chronic inflammation produced by high saturated fat intake can also lead to insulin resistance, a condition where the body's cells do not respond properly to insulin. Insulin resistance is a precursor to type 2 diabetes and is connected with obesity, metabolic syndrome, and cardiovascular disease. Reducing saturated fat consumption can help increase insulin sensitivity and lessen the risk of certain diseases.

Fried Foods and Digestive Issues

Fried foods are a popular component of many diets, but their high fat content and technique of preparation can contribute to different stomach disorders. Consuming fried meals often can contribute to gastrointestinal discomfort, as well as more serious digestive diseases.

Gastrointestinal Discomfort: Fried meals are often heavy in harmful fats and can be difficult to digest. The high-fat content might slow down the digestion process, resulting in symptoms such as bloating, gas, and stomach cramps. This can be particularly troublesome for those with digestive diseases such as irritable bowel syndrome (IBS) or acid reflux, as fried meals can increase their symptoms.

Gallbladder Stress: The gallbladder plays a critical function in processing lipids by producing bile in the digestive system. Consuming significant amounts of fried meals can place additional stress on the gallbladder, perhaps leading to the production of gallstones or inflammation of the gallbladder (cholecystitis). This might cause serious discomfort and necessitate medical care.

Pancreatitis: Pancreatitis is an inflammation of the pancreas that can be induced by a high-fat diet. The pancreas generates enzymes that assist digest fats, but ingesting excessive amounts of fried meals can cause these enzymes to become hyperactive and harm the pancreas. Symptoms of pancreatitis include intense stomach pain, nausea, and vomiting, and the disease can be life-threatening if not treated swiftly.

Increased Risk of Cancer: Some studies have revealed a relationship between heavy intake of fried meals and an increased risk of certain forms of cancer, such as colorectal and breast cancer. This may be related to the development of hazardous chemicals, such as acrylamide and advanced glycation end products (AGEs), during the frying process. These chemicals can induce oxidative stress and DNA damage, leading to the development of cancer.

Healthier Fat Choices

In the context of a balanced diet, not all fats are created equal. While some forms of fat can contribute to numerous health difficulties, others are vital for sustaining healthy bodily processes. Making healthy fat choices entails knowing the types of fats available and how they affect health. This section discusses the many kinds of fats and highlights the healthier ones that should be preferred.

Monounsaturated Fats: These fats are considered heart-healthy and may be found in a range of meals. Monounsaturated fats can help reduce harmful cholesterol levels in the blood, which can minimize the risk of heart disease and stroke. They also give nutrients that help create and maintain the body's cells. Common sources of monounsaturated fats include:

Olive Oil: A mainstay in the Mediterranean diet, olive oil is high in monounsaturated fats and has been linked to several health advantages, including decreased inflammation and a lower risk of chronic illnesses.

Avocados: Avocados are filled with monounsaturated fats and also give fiber, vitamins, and minerals.

Polyunsaturated Fats: These fats are necessary, meaning the body cannot generate them and they must be received via the diet. Polyunsaturated fats contain omega-3 and omega-6 fatty acids, which are needed for brain function and cell development. Sources of polyunsaturated fats include:

Fatty Fish: Salmon, mackerel, sardines, and trout are rich in omega-3 fatty acids, which have anti-inflammatory qualities and enhance heart health.

Flaxseeds and Chia Seeds: Both seeds are great plant-based sources of omega-3 fatty acids and contain fiber and protein.

Walnuts: Walnuts are another fantastic source of omega-3 fatty acids and are helpful for heart health.

Omega-3 Fatty Acids and Their Benefits

Omega-3 fatty acids are a form of polyunsaturated fat that is necessary for different body activities. They are recognized for their strong health advantages, notably in decreasing inflammation and supporting heart and brain function. There are three primary forms of omega-3 fatty acids: ALA (alpha-linolenic acid), DHA (docosahexaenoic acid), and EPA (eicosapentaenoic acid).

Heart Health: Omega-3 fatty acids are well-known for their cardioprotective properties. They help lower blood pressure, reduce triglycerides, minimize the risk of irregular cardiac rhythms, and prevent the creation of arterial plaque. Regular consumption of omega-3-rich meals can considerably lower the risk of heart disease and stroke.

Brain Health: DHA, a form of omega-3 fatty acid, is a fundamental structural component of the brain and retina. Adequate intake of DHA is necessary for brain growth and function. Omega-3 fatty acids have been demonstrated to boost cognitive performance, lower the risk of neurodegenerative illnesses, and support mental health by relieving symptoms of depression and anxiety.

Anti-Inflammatory Properties: Chronic inflammation is a primary cause of many severe illnesses, including heart disease, cancer, and autoimmune disorders. Omega-3 fatty acids offer significant anti-inflammatory properties, which can help minimize the risk of chronic inflammation and its related health concerns.

Eye Health: Omega-3 fatty acids, particularly DHA, are vital for sustaining good eyesight. They help protect against macular degeneration, a primary cause of age-related blindness.

Pregnancy and Child Development: Omega-3 fatty acids are vital for the development of the fetal brain and eyes throughout pregnancy. They also promote the health of the mother, minimizing the risk of premature delivery and increasing general maternal health.

Cooking Methods for Healthier Meals

Choosing healthy fats is simply one component of preparing nutritious meals. The cooking methods utilized can considerably alter the nutritional content of the meal. Here are some healthy cooking methods that conserve nutrients and limit the creation of toxic compounds:

Steaming: Steaming is one of the healthiest cooking methods since it keeps most of the nutrients in vegetables and seafood. It includes heating food with steam from boiling water, which helps retain vitamins and minerals that can be lost through other cooking techniques.

Baking: Baking is a dry-heat cooking method that is good for preparing meat, fish, and vegetables. It requires minimum additional fat and helps retain nutrients. Baking at lower temperatures can help reduce the development of hazardous chemicals that occur at higher temperatures.

Grilling: Grilling may be a healthy cooking method if done correctly. It causes fat to drain away from the meal, decreasing the overall fat level. However, it's vital to prevent charring the food, as this might develop carcinogenic substances. Using marinades and cooking at moderate temperatures can help limit the production of these hazardous chemicals.

Sautéing: Sautéing includes cooking food quickly in a tiny amount of oil over medium-high heat. Using healthy oils like olive or avocado oil can make this procedure a nutritional alternative. Sautéing maintains the texture and flavor of veggies and may be a fantastic way to include healthy fats into meals.

Poaching: Poaching involves cooking food gradually in simmering water or broth. This approach is perfect for delicate goods like fish and eggs. Poaching helps maintain moisture and nutrients without adding more fat.

Slow Cooking: Slow cooking is a handy approach that includes cooking food at a low temperature for an extended period. This approach helps maintain nutrients and enriches the tastes of the components. It's particularly useful for preparing soups, stews, and casseroles.

Roasting: Roasting is a dry-heat cooking method that consist of roasting food in an oven. It's suitable for meats, poultry, and veggies. Roasting at moderate temperatures can help retain nutrients and decrease the production of toxic chemicals.

Stir-Frying: Stir-frying is a rapid cooking method that includes heating food over high heat with a small amount of oil. It's a terrific method to cook veggies while maintaining their nutrients and adding healthy fats. Using a range of colorful veggies and lean meats may make stir-frying a nutritious and balanced dinner choice.

Implementing these healthy cooking methods into your routine can boost the nutritional integrity of your meals while keeping flavor and texture. By making careful decisions regarding the types of fats utilized and the cooking processes employed, you may make tasty, health-promoting recipes that boost overall well-being.

Chapter 7

Dairy Products

Dairy products, including milk, cheese, yogurt, and butter, are a mainstay in many cuisines across the world. They are acclaimed for their strong nutritional value, notably their high quantities of calcium, protein, and vitamins such as vitamin D and B12. However, the link between dairy intake and health is nuanced and varied. While dairy may be a healthy element of a balanced diet, it also has the potential to affect hormonal health and skin disorders, such as acne, in important ways.

Dairy and Hormonal Health

Hormones serve a key role in regulating many biological processes, and the foods we consume can alter our hormonal balance. Dairy products, for example, include a range of hormones, both naturally occurring and those added during the production process. This includes estrogens, progesterone, and other growth hormones, which might impact the body's endocrine system.

What a Dairy Affects Estrogen Levels

Estrogen is a critical hormone in the female reproductive system, and maintaining its balance is essential for general health. Dairy products, especially those from cows treated with growth hormones, can contain high quantities of estrogen and other hormone-like compounds. When eaten, these hormones can enter the human body and alter its hormonal equilibrium.

Endogenous Estrogens: Cows naturally make estrogen, and these hormones can be present in the milk they produce. High amounts of endogenous estrogens in dairy products can contribute to increased estrogen consumption in humans, which may upset the normal hormonal balance, particularly in women. This disturbance can appear in different ways, including menstrual abnormalities and an increased risk of hormone-related illnesses such as breast cancer.

Added Hormones: In some dairy farming procedures, cows are injected with synthetic hormones to improve milk output. These additional hormones can further boost the hormone levels in dairy products, exacerbating their influence on human health.

Impact on Estrogen Metabolism: Consumption of dairy can also impact how the body metabolizes estrogen. Some research shows that an increased dairy diet might affect the ratio of estrogen metabolites, potentially raising the amounts of more strong and dangerous estrogen forms. This imbalance in metabolism may lead to illnesses such as endometriosis and polycystic ovarian syndrome (PCOS).

Links Between Dairy and Acne

Acne is a widespread skin disorder that affects millions of individuals worldwide, and its association with food, particularly dairy consumption, has been the focus of much research. Several studies have proven a relationship between dairy products and the worsening of acne symptoms.

Hormonal Influence: As previously discussed, dairy products include hormones that might alter the body's endocrine system. These hormones, notably androgens and insulin-like growth factor 1 (IGF-1), can encourage the creation of sebum, the greasy material that can clog pores and contribute to acne. Increased levels of IGF-1, which is naturally present in milk and can be enhanced by dairy consumption, have been connected with greater sebum production and more severe acne.

Inflammatory Response: Dairy products can provoke inflammatory reactions in the body. Inflammation is a significant element in the development of acne, and ingesting foods that cause inflammation can aggravate acne symptoms. Some individuals may have a sensitivity or allergy to dairy, which can further intensify the inflammatory response and aggravate skin issues.

Glycemic Load: Dairy products, especially those with added sugars such as flavored yogurts and sweetened milk, can have a high glycemic load. Foods having a high glycemic index can produce fast rises in blood sugar levels, leading to increased insulin production. Elevated insulin levels can, in turn, encourage the production of androgens and IGF-1, both of which are connected to the development and severity of acne.

Types of Dairies and Acne: Different types of dairy products may have varied effects on acne. For example, skim milk has been found to have a greater connection with acne compared to full milk. This may be owing to the larger quantity of bioavailable hormones and proteins in skim milk, which can impact acne development more dramatically.

Dairy Products and Nutritional Value

While there are issues surrounding the hormonal influence of dairy products, it is crucial to appreciate their nutritional advantages. Dairy is a great source of vital nutrients that help to overall health, including:

Calcium: Dairy products are one of the finest dietary sources of calcium, which is vital for keeping healthy bones and teeth. Adequate calcium consumption is vital for avoiding osteoporosis and promoting appropriate bone formation.

Protein: Dairy products contain high-quality protein, which is vital for muscle repair, development, and general body processes. Proteins in dairy include all necessary amino acids, making them a complete protein source.

Vitamins and Minerals: In addition to calcium, dairy products are rich in vitamins D, B12, and riboflavin, as well as minerals such as phosphorus and potassium. These nutrients serve critical roles in energy generation, neuron function, and sustaining general health.

Dairy Alternatives

Dairy substitutes have gained popularity in recent years, spurred by numerous causes including health concerns, ethical issues, and dietary choices. These alternatives, which span a wide range of plant-based products, offer options for persons looking to decrease or remove dairy from their diets. From plant-based milk to non-dairy cheeses, the market for dairy substitutes continues to develop, offering customers choices that appeal to various tastes and nutritional demands.

Plant-Based Milk and Cheese

Plant-Based Milk: Plant-based milk, such as almond milk, soy milk, coconut milk, and oat milk, have developed as popular alternatives to cow's milk. These milks are often created by soaking and combining different plant materials with water, then straining to form a liquid-like ordinary milk. Each form of plant-based milk has diverse tastes, textures, and nutritional profiles, making them appropriate for varied culinary purposes and dietary requirements.

Almond Milk: Almond milk is produced from ground almonds and water, frequently supplemented with vitamins and minerals including calcium and vitamin D. It has a nutty flavor and creamy texture, making it a flexible choice for drinking, cooking, and baking. Almond milk is naturally low in calories and carbs, making it a popular option for people seeking a lighter alternative to dairy milk.

Soy Milk: Soy milk is created from soybeans and water, delivering a creamy texture and a mild, slightly nutty flavor. It is one of the most nutritionally equivalent alternatives to cow's milk, sometimes supplemented with calcium, vitamin D, and B12. Soy milk is a complete protein source, including all essential amino acids, making it an acceptable alternative for vegetarians and vegans.

Coconut Milk: Coconut milk is created from the flesh of ripe coconuts mixed with water. It has a luscious, creamy texture and a mild coconut taste. Coconut milk is richer in fat compared to other plant-based milk, offering a supply of medium-chain triglycerides (MCTs) which are considered to give different health advantages. It is widely used in curries, sweets, and smoothies.

Oat Milk: Oat milk is created from oats mixed with water and filtered. It has a mild, somewhat sweet flavor and a creamy mouthfeel, comparable to cow's milk. Oat milk is typically fortified with elements such as calcium and vitamin D, making it a healthful alternative for people wishing to enhance their consumption of these critical nutrients.

Non-Dairy Cheese: Non-dairy cheeses have progressed dramatically in recent years, giving alternatives to typical cheese manufactured from animal milk. These cheeses are often manufactured from plant-based materials such as nuts, seeds, soy, or coconut oil. While they may not precisely match the flavor and texture of dairy cheese, they give possibilities for consumers seeking dairy-free alternatives.

Nut-Based Cheeses: Cheeses produced from nuts such as cashews, almonds, or macadamias are popular choices among plant-based diners. These cheeses are often made by combining soaked nuts with probiotics or enzymes for fermentation, resulting in a creamy, tangy cheese-like product. Nut-based cheeses can be aged and seasoned to imitate many forms of dairy cheese.

Soy-Based Cheeses: Soy-based cheeses are generally created using fermented soybeans combined with oils and spices to create a cheese-like texture and flavor. These cheeses may melt and stretch like typical dairy cheese, making them excellent for cooking and topping foods.

Coconut Oil-Based Cheeses: Cheeses manufactured from coconut oil are another choice for dairy-free customers. These cheeses are frequently manufactured to melt and have a creamy feel, comparable to dairy cheese. They may be utilized in both savory and sweet recipes, allowing diversity in culinary applications.

Nutritional Comparison of Dairy vs. Non-Dairy

Nutritional Content: When comparing dairy and non-dairy alternatives, there are noteworthy changes in nutritional makeup. Dairy milk is recognized for its high calcium content, which is vital for bone development and general growth. It also contains considerable amounts of protein and vital vitamins such as vitamin D and B12. However, dairy milk can be rich in saturated fats and cholesterol, which may be a problem for those with certain health issues.

Calcium: Many plant-based milks are fortified with calcium to meet or exceed the calcium level of dairy milk. For example, soy milk and almond milk can have identical quantities of calcium when fortified. Calcium-fortified plant-based milk is vital for persons who rely on dairy for their calcium intake.

Protein: Dairy milk is a complete protein source, meaning it provides all nine essential amino acids necessary for human health. Plant-based milk differs in protein concentration, with soy milk being the closest in protein content to dairy milk. Other plant-based milks may be lower in protein unless fortified.

Fat Content: Dairy milk includes various quantities of fat depending on the kind (whole, reduced-fat, skim). Whole dairy milk is richer in saturated fats, whereas reduced-fat and skim versions have lower fat content. Plant-based milks often have reduced saturated fat content and may contain beneficial fats such as monounsaturated and polyunsaturated fats.

Vitamins and Minerals: Both dairy and non-dairy alternatives can be fortified with key vitamins and minerals to boost their nutritional value. Fortification generally contains vitamin D, vitamin B12, and sometimes vitamin A and riboflavin. This guarantees that non-dairy alternatives supply identical nutrients to those naturally found in dairy milk.

Dairy substitutes provide a varied selection of solutions for persons wishing to decrease or remove dairy from their diets. From plant-based milks like almond, soy, coconut, and oat milk to non-dairy cheeses produced from nuts, seeds, and soy, these options appeal to diverse dietary choices and nutritional demands. While dairy products supply critical nutrients like calcium and protein, dairy replacements can offer equivalent nutritional advantages with lower amounts of saturated fats and cholesterol. Understanding the nutritional distinctions between dairy and non-dairy products allows consumers to make educated decisions that match their health objectives and dietary preferences. Whether for health reasons, ethical considerations, or taste preferences, dairy replacements continue to play a key part in current dietary habits, giving viable choices for individuals wishing to vary their diets while preserving nutritional sufficiency.

Chapter 8

Salty Foods and Bloating

Bloating is a frequent discomfort defined by a sense of fullness and tightness in the belly. Salty meals can considerably contribute to bloating, which is a typical pain. The collection of gas or fluid in the gastrointestinal system is a common cause of bloating, and the ingestion of foods that are high in salt can make this problem even worse. Understanding the relationship between bloating and salty foods may assist individuals in making better choices regarding their diet, which can help them feel less uncomfortable and enhance their overall health.

Sodium and Water Retention

In addition to its involvement in maintaining fluid equilibrium, neuronal function, and muscular contraction, sodium is an important mineral that plays a key part in these processes. However, consuming an excessive amount of salt can cause water retention, which in turn adds to bloating at the same time. When the body takes in an excessive amount of sodium, it makes up for it by retaining water to reduce the amount of sodium that is present in the bloodstream. To maintain this process, the kidneys are responsible for regulating the quantity of salt and water that is eliminated through the urine.

Water retention, or edema, happens when excess fluid collects in the body's tissues, resulting in swelling and puffiness, mainly in the hands, feet, and belly. The accumulation of fluid can lead to bloating and pain, resulting in a feeling of distention and tightness in the abdominal region. Through the process of allowing the body to empty extra fluid and restore equilibrium, reducing the amount of sodium that is consumed can help reduce these symptoms.

The Science Behind Bloating

Bloating is a multidimensional disorder that can originate from different reasons, including nutrition, lifestyle, and underlying medical issues. The science of bloating includes the interaction of numerous physiological systems, including gas generation, fluid retention, and digestive function.

Gas Production: One of the main reasons for bloating is the production of gas in the gastrointestinal system. This can occur when undigested food is fermented by microorganisms in the large intestine, creating gases such as carbon dioxide, methane, and hydrogen. High-fiber diets, fizzy beverages, and certain carbohydrates can lead to increased gas production.

Fluid Retention: As discussed previously, high salt consumption can lead to fluid retention, which adds to bloating. Hormonal variations, particularly in women throughout the menstrual cycle, can significantly impact fluid balance and induce bloating.

Digestive Function: Impaired digestion or delayed gastrointestinal motility can lead to the accumulation of gas and fluid in the digestive tract, producing bloating. Conditions such as irritable bowel syndrome (IBS), small intestinal bacterial overgrowth (SIBO), and constipation can aggravate bloating by interrupting normal digestive processes.

Gut Microbiota: The gut microbiota, the varied population of bacteria dwelling in the digestive system, plays a key role in digestion and general health. An imbalance in gut flora can contribute to increased gas production and bloating. Probiotics and a balanced diet can help maintain healthy gut bacteria and minimize bloating.

High-Sodium Foods to Avoid

To control bloating efficiently, it is vital to identify and limit high-sodium meals in the diet. Here are some frequent origins of high sodium:

Processed Foods: Many processed foods, including canned soups, frozen dinners, and packaged snacks, include high quantities of salt as a preservative and taste enhancer. Reading nutrition labels and choosing low-sodium choices can help minimize salt consumption.

Fast Food: Fast food and restaurant meals are generally high in sodium due to the usage of salt and sodium-containing additives. Opting for prepared meals or picking lower-sodium menu items can help decrease salt consumption.

Deli Meats and Sausages: Processed meats such as ham, bacon, salami, and sausages are often heavy in salt. Reducing consumption of these meats and picking lower-sodium alternatives can help decrease overall salt intake.

Cheese and Dairy Products: Some cheeses and dairy products, notably processed cheese and cheese spreads, contain substantial quantities of salt. Choosing fresh or low-sodium cheese kinds might be advantageous.

Condiments and Sauces: Condiments such as soy sauce, ketchup, mustard, and salad dressings can contain high quantities of salt. Using herbs, spices, and homemade dressings helps minimize salt consumption.

Snack Foods: Chips, pretzels, popcorn, and other salty snacks are substantial sources of sodium. Choosing unsalted or mildly salted versions of these foods might help decrease sodium consumption.

Bread and Baked Goods: Many varieties of bread, rolls, and baked goods include additional salt. Opting for whole-grain or low-sodium bread alternatives helps lower salt intake.

Practical Tips for Reducing Sodium Intake

Reducing salt consumption needs intentional effort and thoughtful eating habits. Here are some practical strategies to help manage and minimize salt consumption:

Read Nutrition Labels: Checking nutrition labels for salt levels can help identify high-sodium meals. Intention to pick items with reduced sodium levels or labeled as "low-sodium" or "no added salt."

Rinse Canned goods: Rinsing canned goods such as beans and vegetables might help eliminate some of the extra salt. Alternatively, choosing "no salt added" or "low-sodium" versions of canned items might be advantageous.

Limit Processed and Packaged Foods: Reducing the consumption of processed and packaged foods can dramatically cut salt intake. Opting for fresh, nutritious meals such as fruits, vegetables, lean meats, and whole grains will boost overall health and prevent bloating.

Choose Low-Sodium Alternatives: Numerous food products have low-sodium alternatives available. Selecting these alternatives can assist limit salt consumption without compromising flavor.

Be Mindful When Dining Out: When eating out, ask for meals to be made with less salt, and pick dishes that are naturally lower in sodium. Avoiding sauces and dressings or getting them on the side can also aid to decrease salt consumption.

Managing Sodium Intake

Sodium is a vital element for maintaining fluid equilibrium, neuron function, and muscle contraction. However, high salt intake can lead to several health concerns, including hypertension, cardiovascular disease, and bloating. Managing salt consumption is vital for sustaining overall health and well-being. This entails recognizing the sources of sodium in the diet, monitoring daily intake, and adopting informed dietary choices to decrease excess salt consumption.

Tips for Reducing Salt in Your Diet

Reducing salt in your diet doesn't imply sacrificing flavor. With a few easy tweaks and conscious eating habits, you may dramatically cut your salt consumption and still enjoy tasty meals. Here are a handful of practical strategies for lowering salt in your diet:

Read Nutrition Labels: The first step to reducing sodium consumption is to become aware of how much salt is in the items you eat. Check nutrition labels for salt amount per serving, and seek for goods with lower sodium levels. A daily consumption of less than 2,300 milligrams of salt is suggested for most individuals, with an optimal limit of 1,500 mg for those with hypertension or at risk for cardiovascular illnesses.

Choose Fresh Over Processed Foods: Processed and packaged foods are generally high in sodium, as salt is employed as a preservative and taste enhancer. Opt for fresh, healthy foods whenever feasible. Fresh fruits, vegetables, lean meats, and whole grains are naturally low in sodium and deliver critical nutrients without extra salt.

Cook at Home: Preparing meals at home helps you to manage the quantity of salt used. usage of fresh ingredients and control the usage of processed meals. When cooking, consider minimizing the quantity of salt in dishes and add herbs, spices, and other flavorings instead.

Rinse Canned Foods: If you use canned veggies, beans, or other canned items, rinse them under water to eliminate some of the additional salt. Choose "nor salt added" or "low-sodium" variants whenever feasible.

Use Salt replacements Wisely: Salt replacements might be an alternative for people trying to limit salt consumption. However, be cautious with alternatives that include potassium chloride, especially if you have renal concerns or are on medicine that impacts potassium levels. Always contact a healthcare expert before utilizing salt replacements.

Monitor Portion Sizes: Larger servings might lead to greater salt consumption. Be cautious of portion sizes and aim to stay within the suggested serving sizes to help limit salt consumption.

Flavorful, Low-Sodium Alternatives

Cutting back on salt doesn't mean your meals have to be boring. Various delectable, low-sodium options may enhance the taste of your food without adding excessive salt. Here are some tips for making your meals pleasant and healthy:

Citrus Juices and Zests: Lemon, lime, and orange juices and zests may provide a bright, tangy taste to salads, marinades, and cooked foods. The acidity of citrus fruits can help enhance other tastes, decreasing the need for extra salt.

Vinegar: Various varieties of vinegar, such as balsamic, apple cider, red wine, and rice vinegar, may give depth and richness to your dishes. Use vinegar in dressings, marinades, or as a finishing touch for vegetables and meats.

Garlic and Onions: Fresh garlic and onions offer a strong taste to recipes. Sautéed, roasted, or raw, these fragrant vegetables may enhance the taste of soups, stews, sauces, and salads.

Fresh Herbs: Basil, cilantro, parsley, dill, and mint are just a few examples of fresh herbs that may add bright flavors to your dishes. Use them abundantly in salads, sauces, soups, and garnishes.

Spices: A broad assortment of spices can substitute salt in your cooking. Experiment with spices like cumin, coriander, turmeric, paprika, chili powder, and cinnamon to add new tastes to your food.

Pepper and Pepper Flakes: Black pepper and red pepper flakes may lend a spicy touch to your food. They are ideal for flavoring meats, veggies, and pasta recipes.

Nutritional Yeast: This savory, cheesy-tasting ingredient is low in sodium and may be used to flavor popcorn, pasta, veggies, and sauces. It is also rich in vitamins and minerals, making it a beneficial addition to your diet.

Low-Sodium Broths: When creating soups, stews, or sauces, use low-sodium or homemade broths to limit the sodium content. Homemade broths may be created using fresh ingredients and can be frozen for later use.

No-Salt Seasoning Mixes: Many businesses provide no-salt seasoning mixes that incorporate various herbs and spices. These can be handy for adding taste without increasing salt.

Fermented Foods: Foods like kimchi, sauerkraut, and miso may give a sour, umami taste to recipes without the need for more salt. Be careful of the salt concentration in some fermented foods, and pick low-sodium choices where available.

Chapter 9

Alcohol and Menstrual Health

Alcohol consumption is a regular aspect of social gatherings and relaxation routines for many people. However, its impacts on menstrual health are generally disregarded. Alcohol can alter numerous aspects of the menstrual cycle, including hormone levels, cycle regularity, and the severity of premenstrual symptoms. Understanding how alcohol impacts menstruation health is vital for women wanting to manage their periods and preserve overall well-being.

Alcohol can disturb the hormonal balance, which is needed for a regular menstrual cycle. Hormones such as estrogen and progesterone play crucial roles in regulating the menstrual cycle, and alcohol intake can change their levels. For instance, studies have shown that alcohol can raise estrogen levels, which might lead to hormonal abnormalities. This imbalance can produce irregular periods, increase menstrual bleeding, and enhance premenstrual syndrome (PMS) symptoms, such as mood swings, breast pain, and bloating.

Furthermore, drinking can increase PMS symptoms. Women who consume alcohol may have more severe mood fluctuations, anxiety, and depression during their menstrual cycle. Alcohol's depressing effects on the central nervous system might worsen emotional symptoms associated with PMS. Additionally, alcohol's diuretic qualities can lead to dehydration, which can increase physical symptoms including headaches, lethargy, and bloating.

Alcohol's Impact on the Body

The effects of alcohol on the body are diverse, involving many organs and systems. When taken, alcohol is quickly absorbed into the bloodstream through the stomach and small intestine. It subsequently flows to the liver, where it is processed. The liver can digest a limited quantity of alcohol at a time, therefore excessive intake leads to the accumulation of alcohol in the blood, damaging the brain and other organs.

One of the principal impacts of alcohol on the body is its impact on the central nervous system. Alcohol operates as a depressive, slowing down brain activity and weakening cognitive and motor skills. This can result in slurred speech, impaired judgment, and diminished coordination. Over time, chronic alcohol drinking can lead to long-term cognitive deficits and neurological damage.

Alcohol also affects the cardiovascular system. While moderate alcohol use has been connected with certain cardiovascular benefits, such as increased levels of "good" HDL cholesterol, excessive drinking can lead to major health complications. Heavy alcohol usage can increase blood pressure, induce cardiomyopathy (a condition of the heart muscle), and elevate the risk of stroke. Additionally, alcohol can contribute to an abnormal heartbeat, known as arrhythmia.

The liver is particularly sensitive to the effects of alcohol. Chronic alcohol intake can induce several liver illnesses, including fatty liver, alcoholic hepatitis, fibrosis, and cirrhosis. The liver's primary role is to detoxify the body, but excessive alcohol intake can overwhelm this mechanism, leading to liver damage and inflammation.

Effects on Sleep and Hydration

Alcohol has a substantial impact on sleep and hydration, both of which are crucial for general wellness. While alcohol may initially assist some people fall asleep faster, it impairs the quality of sleep. Alcohol interferes with the regular sleep cycle, particularly the rapid eye movement (REM) stage, which is necessary for restorative sleep and cognitive performance.

After consuming alcohol, individuals generally experience interrupted sleep, frequent awakenings, and difficulties staying asleep. This interruption in the sleep cycle can contribute to daytime weariness, poor focus, and diminished memory. Over time, poor sleep quality can have major health repercussions, including reduced immune function, weight gain, and an increased risk of chronic illnesses like diabetes and heart disease.

Hydration is another crucial aspect affected by alcohol usage. Alcohol is a diuretic, meaning it stimulates urine output and leads to fluid loss. This diuretic effect might result in dehydration, characterized by symptoms such as dry mouth, thirst, headache, and dizziness. Dehydration can also increase the effects of a hangover, including weariness, nausea, and irritability.

In addition to its diuretic qualities, alcohol can interfere with the body's ability to manage water and electrolyte balance. This disruption can lead to an imbalance in electrolytes such as sodium, potassium, and magnesium, which are required for appropriate muscle function, nerve transmission, and hydration.

Alcohol and Menstrual Cramps

Menstrual cramps, or dysmenorrhea, are a frequent and often debilitating symptom experienced by many women during their menstrual cycle. These cramps are generated by the contraction of the uterine muscles, prompted by the production of prostaglandins, which are hormone-like chemicals implicated in pain and inflammation.

Alcohol can influence the severity of menstrual cramps in numerous ways.

Firstly, alcohol's inflammatory properties might worsen the pain associated with menstrual cramps. Alcohol consumption can enhance the production of inflammatory prostaglandins, resulting in more powerful uterine contractions and pain. Women who consume alcohol may have harsher and longer menstrual cramps compared to those who abstain.

Moreover, alcohol's dehydrating effect might also contribute to the severity of period cramps. Dehydration can cause muscles to cramp and spasm more easily, including the uterine muscles. Ensuring appropriate hydration is vital for decreasing the discomfort associated with menstrual cramps, and alcohol's diuretic effects might hinder this effort.

In addition to its inflammatory and drying effects, alcohol can hinder the body's capacity to absorb and utilize key nutrients that are crucial for treating period cramps. For instance, magnesium is a mineral recognized for its muscle-relaxing qualities, and it can help ease period cramps. However, alcohol use might interfere with magnesium absorption, potentially leading to a shortfall and aggravating cramps.

Alcohol's Broader Effects on Women's Health

Beyond its impact on menstruation health, alcohol intake can have larger ramifications for women's health. Women generally have a lesser tolerance for alcohol compared to men, due to variations in body composition and metabolism. Women tend to have a higher amount of body fat and lower quantities of the enzyme alcohol dehydrogenase, which is responsible for breaking down alcohol in the stomach. This means that women absorb more alcohol into their bloodstream and metabolize it more slowly, leading to higher blood alcohol concentrations and greater vulnerability to alcohol-related health concerns.

One noteworthy issue is the increased risk of breast cancer linked with alcohol intake. Research has indicated that even moderate alcohol drinking can boost the risk of breast cancer in women. Alcohol can increase estrogen levels, which may encourage the growth of hormone-receptor-positive breast tumors. Women with a family history of breast cancer or other risk factors should be extremely cautious about their alcohol usage.

Alcohol can also damage bone health, which is particularly significant for women due to the higher risk of osteoporosis. Chronic alcohol intake can interfere with the balance of calcium and vitamin D, critical elements for bone health. This can lead to diminished bone density and an increased risk of fractures.

Reducing Alcohol Consumption

Reducing alcohol use is a vital step for many individuals aiming to enhance their health and well-being. Whether driven by health concerns, a desire for improved sleep, or an interest in boosting general quality of life, cutting back on alcohol can bring various benefits. It's crucial to approach this objective with a plan that includes practical techniques and alternatives to assure success and sustainability.

One of the key motives for minimizing alcohol intake is the enormous influence it has on overall health. Excessive drinking is connected to a plethora of health difficulties, including liver disease, cardiovascular problems, and an increased risk of some cancers. Moreover, drinking can negatively affect mental health, contributing to anxiety, depression, and poor cognitive performance. By limiting intake, individuals can decrease these hazards and promote improved physical and mental health.

Additionally, cutting back on alcohol can enhance sleep quality. While alcohol may initially assist some people fall asleep, it disturbs the sleep cycle, leading to poor-quality rest. Reducing alcohol consumption can help restore natural sleep patterns, resulting in more restful and refreshing sleep. This can lead to greater mood, enhanced cognitive function, and overall improved everyday performance.

Strategies for Cutting Back

Reducing alcohol use takes a careful strategy, especially for people who have integrated drinking into their social routines or use it as a coping technique. Here are numerous successful techniques for cutting back:

Set Clear Goals: Start by setting clear, quantifiable goals for limiting alcohol intake. Whether it's restricting the number of drinks per week or choosing specific days to abstain, having defined aims can provide direction and incentive.

Track Your Drinking: Keeping a record of when and how much you drink can help you become more conscious of your consumption patterns. This awareness might be the first step toward making substantial changes.

Plan Alcohol-Free Days: Select specific days of the week as alcohol-free. This can help break the habit of everyday drinking and allow your body to recuperate from any previous alcohol intake.

Drink Slowly: When you do choose to drink, do it slowly. Sipping your drink and taking breaks between sips can limit the overall amount you consume and allow you to enjoy the beverage without overindulging.

Eat Before and During Drinking: Consuming food might reduce the absorption of alcohol into your system, decreasing its influence. Opt for a balanced lunch before drinking and healthy snacks during.

Avoid Triggers: Identify circumstances, places, or people that trigger your desire to drink and identify techniques to control or avoid these triggers. For instance, if social gatherings are a trigger, organize activities that don't focus on alcohol.

Find Alternatives: Replace alcoholic beverages with non-alcoholic ones. This can help you keep the ritual of having a drink without the bad effects of alcohol.

Seek Support: Talk to friends, relatives, or a healthcare professional about your aim to minimize alcohol use. Support from others can bring encouragement and accountability.

Engage in New Pastimes: Find new hobbies or pastimes that don't entail drinking. Physical activities, creative endeavors, or volunteering might create a sense of fulfillment and minimize the temptation to drink.

Practice Mindfulness: Mindfulness and stress-reduction activities, such as meditation or yoga, can help manage the emotional triggers that often lead to drinking.

Non-Alcoholic Drink Options

Exploring non-alcoholic drink options is a terrific approach to limiting alcohol intake while still enjoying delectable and refreshing beverages. The market for non-alcoholic drinks has increased tremendously, offering a wide range of choices that appeal to varied tastes and preferences. Here are some common non-alcoholic drink options:

Sparkling Water: Sparkling water is a diverse and refreshing alternative. It comes in several flavors and can be consumed on its own or with a dash of fruit juice for extra flavor. Brands like LaCroix, Perrier, and San Pellegrino offer a variety of possibilities.

Non-Alcoholic Beer: For beer fans, non-alcoholic beers provide the taste of regular beer without the alcohol. Many breweries now provide high-quality non-alcoholic beers that resemble the flavor and scent of their alcoholic counterparts. Popular brands include Heineken 0.0, Athletic Brewing Co., and Clausthaler.

Mocktails: Mocktails are non-alcoholic adaptations of traditional cocktails. They can be made at home or ordered at pubs and restaurants. Some popular mocktails include virgin mojitos, non-alcoholic margaritas, and alcohol-free piña coladas. These beverages frequently employ fresh fruit juices, herbs, and sparkling water to create complex and delicious flavors.

Kombucha: Kombucha is a fermented tea beverage that is naturally carbonated and slightly sour. It contains probiotics, which might be useful for intestinal health. Kombucha comes in numerous tastes, and many manufacturers offer choices with low or no added sugar. Some popular brands are GT's, Health-Ade, and Brew Dr.

Fresh Juices and Smoothies: Freshly squeezed juices and smoothies made from fruits and vegetables are wholesome and delicious alternatives. They can be tailored to suitable personal preferences and dietary concerns. For a pleasant drink, try a blend of citrus fruits, berries, and greens.

Coconut Water: Coconut water is a hydrating and naturally sweet beverage that is high in electrolytes. It's an excellent alternative for staying hydrated, especially after vigorous exertion. Look for brands that offer pure coconut water without additional sweeteners.

Infused Water: Infusing water with fresh fruits, vegetables, and herbs can enhance flavor without any extra calories or sugars. Popular combos include cucumber and mint, lemon and lime, or berries and basil. Infused water is easy to prepare and may be kept in the refrigerator for a pleasant drink throughout the day.

Non-Alcoholic Wine: For wine aficionados, non-alcoholic wines give a similar experience to traditional wine without the alcohol component. These wines are manufactured by eliminating the alcohol from the wine using various procedures, keeping the flavor and aroma. Some brands to try include Fre, Ariel, and St. Regis.

Plant-Based Milk: Plant-based milk, such as almond, soy, oat, and coconut milk, can be used to produce delightful and creamy beverages. They can be consumed on their own or used as a base for smoothies, lattes, or hot chocolate.

Chapter 10:

Foods that May Cause Digestive Discomfort Common Culprits

Digestive discomfort is a frequent condition that can be altered by varied dietary choices. Certain foods are known to produce bloating, gas, and other forms of digestive irritation. Understanding these common factors can help individuals make informed decisions about their diet and manage symptoms more successfully.

One of the primary offenders is high-fat foods. Foods high in lipids, such as fried foods, fatty cuts of meat, and creamy sauces, can slow down digestion, resulting in bloating and discomfort. These foods take longer to break down, causing them to linger in the digestive tract and generate gas.

Another key category is high-fiber foods, particularly when ingested in big quantities or by those who are not acclimated to a high-fiber diet. While fiber is vital for digestive health, certain types, such as those found in beans, lentils, and certain vegetables like broccoli and Brussels sprouts, can cause excessive gas when they ferment in the intestines.

Dairy products are another typical cause of stomach discomfort, especially for persons who are lactose intolerant. Lactose, the sugar contained in milk, can be difficult to digest for persons who lack the enzyme lactase. It leads to symptoms such as bloating, gas, and diarrhea.

Artificial sweeteners, particularly sugar alcohols like sorbitol and mannitol, are also known to induce stomach difficulties. These sweeteners are not fully absorbed by the body, leading to fermentation by bacteria in the gut, which creates gas and can cause bloating.

Gluten, a protein found in wheat, barley, and rye, can cause stomach discomfort for persons with celiac disease or gluten sensitivity. Symptoms include bloating, gas, and stomach pain. Even those without these issues could find that gluten-containing foods might be burdensome on their digestive tract.

Cruciferous plants, such as cabbage, cauliflower, and kale, are healthy but can induce gas and bloating due to their high level of raffinose, a type of carbohydrate that is not easily digested until it reaches the large intestine, where it is fermented by bacteria.

Carbonated beverages, including soda and sparkling water, introduce extra air into the digestive tract, resulting in belching, bloating, and gas. Similarly, sipping through a straw or chewing gum might also lead you to swallow air, contributing to the same sensations.

Lastly, certain fruits like apples, pears, and prunes might induce digestive discomfort because they contain high quantities of fructose and sorbitol, both of which can be difficult for certain people to digest.

Gas Before Your Period: Why It Happens

Premenstrual gas is a frequent and often painful condition experienced by many individuals. Understanding why it happens can provide insight into how to manage and alleviate this issue.

Causes of Premenstrual Gas

The primary cause of premenstrual gas is hormonal imbalances. In the days preceding a menstrual period, levels of progesterone and estrogen fluctuate substantially. Progesterone, in particular, can cause the smooth muscles of the gastrointestinal system to relax, resulting in slower digestion and increased gas production. This relaxation provides more time for gas to build up and produces bloating and discomfort.

Water retention is another mechanism leading to premenstrual gas. Hormonal changes can cause the body to retain more water, which can make the stomach feel fuller and more bloated. This can worsen the impression of gas and discomfort.

Dietary changes during the premenstrual time can also have a role. Many individuals develop cravings for high-carbohydrate, high-fat, or sugary foods during this time, which can lead to stomach distress and increased gas production. Additionally, these foods can trigger more fermentation in the intestines, leading to increased gas.

Stress and worry, which can be heightened in the premenstrual phase, also influence digestion. The gut is particularly susceptible to stress, and increased anxiety can lead to alterations in gut motility and gas output.

Why Premenstrual Gas Smells

The smell of premenstrual gas can be ascribed to the meals consumed and the bacteria present in the gut. When food is not entirely digested, it goes into the large intestine where microorganisms break it down, creating gasses including methane, hydrogen, and sulfur compounds. Sulfur-containing foods, such as eggs, meat, and certain vegetables, can produce foul-smelling gas when broken down by gut bacteria.

Hormonal shifts can also modify the composition of gut bacteria, perhaps leading to changes in the smell of gas. The mix of bacteria in the gut can alter the types of gases released during digestion.

Remedies for Premenstrual Gassiness

Managing premenstrual gassiness involves a combination of dietary alterations, lifestyle changes, and, if necessary, medicinal measures. Here are some successful remedies:

Dietary Changes: Reducing the intake of high-fat, high-fiber, and sulfur-containing meals in the days coming up to your period can help minimize gas production. Opt for readily digestible foods like lean proteins, white rice, and non-cruciferous veggies.

Smaller, Frequent Meals: Eating smaller, more frequent meals can prevent the digestive system from becoming overwhelmed and lessen the probability of gas buildup.

Hydration: Staying well-hydrated helps maintain normal digestion and can prevent constipation, which can increase gas and bloating. Ought to drink plenty of water throughout the day.

Probiotics: Incorporating probiotics into your diet can help balance gut bacteria and aid digestion. Foods like yogurt, kefir, and fermented vegetables are very good sources of probiotics.

Exercise: Regular physical activity might help accelerate digestion and prevent bloating. Gentle workouts like walking, yoga, or stretching might be particularly beneficial during the premenstrual phase.

Stress Management: Practicing stress-reducing practices such as deep breathing, meditation, and mindfulness can help lessen the impact of stress on your digestive system.

Over-the-Counter Remedies: Simethicone-based treatments like Gas-X can help reduce gas. Additionally, digestive enzymes can aid in the breakdown of difficult-to-digest meals.

Herbal Teas: Certain herbal teas, such as peppermint, ginger, and chamomile, can relax the digestive tract and relieve gas and bloating. These can be specifically useful in the days leading up to your menstruation.

Avoid Carbonated Beverages: Steering clear of soda and other carbonated drinks can help limit the amount of swallowed air and lessen gas production.

Limit Sugar Alcohols: Reducing the intake of sugar alcohols found in sugar-free gum and candies can minimize the gas and bloating they often induce.

Easing Digestive Symptoms

Digestive problems such as bloating, gas, constipation, and diarrhea are typical concerns that can drastically influence one's quality of life. Addressing these symptoms frequently needs a complex approach that includes dietary changes, lifestyle improvements, and even medicinal interventions. Here, we shall study numerous techniques to ease digestive issues efficiently.

One of the key strategies to alleviate digestive issues is by making dietary modifications. Eating smaller, more frequent meals might help prevent the digestive system from becoming overloaded, which can lead to bloating and discomfort. This strategy ensures that the digestive process is smoother and less prone to complications such as gas and bloating.

Hydration plays a critical part in sustaining good digestion. Drinking enough water helps keep the digestive tract lubricated and aids in the transit of food through the intestines. Dehydration can lead to constipation and exacerbate other digestive issues. It is recommended to drink at least eight glasses of water a day, but individual needs may vary based on activity level and climate.

Fiber is vital for digestive health, but it needs to be consumed in the proper amounts and from the right sources. Soluble fiber, found in foods like oats, apples, and carrots, absorbs water and helps form a gel-like substance in the intestines, which can alleviate diarrhea. Insoluble fiber, found in whole grains, nuts, and vegetables, adds volume to the stool and helps avoid constipation. However, increasing fiber intake too soon can contribute to gas and bloating, so it should be done gradually.

Probiotics, the beneficial bacteria found in fermented foods and supplements, can help balance the gut microbiota and enhance digestive health. These microorganisms aid in the digestion of food, absorption of nutrients, and the avoidance of dangerous bacteria overgrowth. Food's rich in probiotics include yogurt, kefir, sauerkraut, kimchi, and miso.

Prebiotics are non-digestible fibers that feed beneficial microorganisms in the gut. They are found in foods like garlic, onions, bananas, and asparagus. Including prebiotics in the diet can boost the growth of probiotics and improve overall gut health.

Regular physical activity is another essential role in alleviating stomach issues. Exercise activates the muscles in the digestive tract, helping to transport food and waste through the system more efficiently. Activities like walking, yoga, and swimming are particularly excellent for digestion.

Stress management is vital for maintaining healthy digestion. The gut is often referred to as the "second brain" because of its sensitivity to stress and emotions. Chronic stress can lead to disorders like irritable bowel syndrome (IBS) and exacerbate other digestive symptoms. Techniques such as deep breathing, meditation, and mindfulness can help reduce stress and enhance digestive health.

Chewing food thoroughly and eating slowly can also improve digestion. This permits the digestive enzymes in saliva to begin breaking down food before it reaches the stomach, lowering the stress on the digestive system and preventing difficulties like gas and bloating.

Beneficial Foods for Gut Health

Maintaining a healthy gut is critical for general well-being since the gut plays a vital role in digestion, nutrition absorption, and immunological function. Incorporating specific items into the diet can boost gut health and help prevent digestive disorders. Here, we will cover numerous foods that are particularly excellent for intestinal health.

Fermented Foods: Fermented foods are rich in probiotics, which are helpful microorganisms that support a healthy gut microbiota. Examples of fermented foods include yogurt, kefir, sauerkraut, kimchi, miso, and kombucha. These foods include live cultures that can help balance the gut microbiota, enhance digestion, and boost immune function. Regular consumption of fermented foods helps alleviate symptoms of digestive diseases such as IBS and diarrhea.

Fiber-Rich Foods: Fiber is vital for maintaining a healthy digestive tract. There are two methods of fiber: soluble and insoluble. Soluble fiber, found in foods like oats, beans, apples, and citrus fruits, helps soften stool and can reduce symptoms of diarrhea. Insoluble fiber, found in whole grains, nuts, and vegetables, provides volume to the stool and can reduce constipation. A diet high in both types of fiber encourages regular bowel motions and a healthy gut.

Leafy Greens: Leafy greens such as spinach, kale, and Swiss chard are rich in fiber, vitamins, and minerals that support intestinal health. They also include chemicals that help feed the beneficial bacteria in the gut, promoting a healthy microbiome. Leafy greens are also abundant in magnesium, which can help ease constipation by relaxing the muscles in the intestines.

Garlic and Onions: Garlic and onions are high in prebiotics, which are non-digestible fibers that feed good gut bacteria. Prebiotics assist increase the number of probiotics in the gut, promoting a healthy microbiome. These foods also contain antibacterial qualities that can help prevent infections in the digestive tract.

Whole Grains: Whole grains such as brown rice, quinoa, barley, and oats are abundant in fiber and minerals they supports gut health. The fiber in whole grains encourages regular bowel motions and helps prevent constipation. Whole grains also include prebiotics that feed good gut microbes.

Apples: Apples are strong in soluble fiber, notably pectin, which helps soften stool and promote regular bowel movements. The fiber in apples also nourishes good gut bacteria and maintains a healthy microbiome.

Apples are also rich in antioxidants that protect the gastrointestinal lining from inflammation and damage.

Bone Broth: Bone broth is rich in gelatin, which can help calm and mend the intestinal lining. It also contains amino acids such as glutamine, which improve intestinal health and reduce inflammation. Drinking bone broth or using it as a foundation for soups and stews can provide several benefits for the digestive system.

Having these nutritious items in the diet can assist promote gut health and prevent digestive disorders. Along with a balanced diet, maintaining a healthy lifestyle that includes regular physical activity, appropriate water, and stress management is vital for optimal digestive health.

Chapter 11

Creating a Balanced Diet Plan

Creating a balanced diet plan entails knowing and incorporating the proper amounts of macronutrients (carbohydrates, proteins, and fats) and micronutrients (vitamins and minerals) to suit the body's needs. A balanced diet ensures that the body gets the vital nutrients required for energy, growth, and overall health.

Macronutrients

Carbohydrates are the body's principal source of energy. They should make up roughly 45-65% of your overall daily calorie consumption. Focus on complex carbs like whole grains, fruits, vegetables, and legumes, which give sustained energy and critical nutrients.

Proteins are necessary for forming and repairing tissues, including muscles, skin, and organs. They should constitute roughly 12-35% of your regular calorie intake. Include a range of protein sources such as lean meats, poultry, fish, eggs, dairy products, legumes, nuts, and seeds.

Fats are important for absorbing fat-soluble vitamins (A, D, E, and K) and generating energy. They should account for roughly 20-35% of your daily calorie consumption. Opt for healthy fats found in avocados, nuts, seeds, olives, and fatty seafood, and limit saturated and trans fats.

Micronutrients

Vitamins and minerals are necessary for different biological activities, including immune support, bone health, and energy production. Ensure a mix of fruits, vegetables, whole grains, and lean proteins to meet these demands.

Hydration

Water is vital for digestion, nutrition absorption, and overall health. Aim for at least 8 cups (2 liters) of water every day, adjusting based on activity level and environment.

Building a Menstrual Health-Friendly Diet

A diet that supports menstruation health should contain items that help control symptoms such as bloating, cramps, and mood swings. This involves focusing on certain nutrients proven to ease menstruation discomfort and boost overall hormonal balance.

Sample Meal Plans and Recipes

To make it practical, here are some meal plans and recipes that contain these critical elements for a balanced diet and menstrual health.

Breakfast Options

Overnight Oats with Berries and Chia Seeds

1/2 cup rolled oats

1/2 cup almond milk

1 tbsp chia seeds

1/2 cup mixed berries

1 tbsp honey

Mix all ingredients in a jar and chill overnight. Top with more berries in the morning.

Spinach and Mushroom Omelette

2 eggs

1 cup spinach

1/2 cup mushrooms, sliced 1 tbsp olive oil

Salt and pepper to taste

Heat olive oil in a skillet, sauté spinach and mushrooms, then add beaten eggs. Cook until eggs are set.

Smoothie Bowl

1 banana

1/2 cup Greek yogurt

1/2 cup spinach

1/2 cup frozen berries

1 tbsp almond butter

Blend all ingredients and top with granola and fresh fruit.

Lunch Options

Quinoa Salad with Avocado and Black Beans

1 cup cooked quinoa

1/2 avocado, diced

1/2 cup black beans, washed

1/2 cup corn

1/4 cup red onion, chopped 1 lime, juiced

Salt and pepper to taste

Mix all ingredients in a bowl and drizzle with lime juice.

Turkey and Veggie Wrap

Whole wheat tortilla

3 slices turkey breast

1/2 cup mixed greens

1/4 cup shredded carrots

1/4 cup sliced cucumber

2 tbsp hummus

Spread hummus on the tortilla, add turkey and vegetables, and roll up.

Lentil Soup

1 cup lentils

1 carrot, diced

1 celery stalk, chopped

1 onion, chopped 2 cloves garlic, minced

4 cups vegetable broth

1 tbsp olive oil

Salt, pepper, and herbs to taste

Sauté vegetables in olive oil, add lentils and stock and cook until lentils are tender.

Dinner Options

Baked Salmon with Quinoa and Steamed Broccoli

1 salmon fillet

1 cup cooked quinoa

1 cup broccoli florets

1 tbsp olive oil

Salt, pepper, and lemon juice to taste

Season salmon with salt, pepper, and lemon juice,
and bake at 400°F for 20 minutes. Serve with quinoa and
steamed broccoli.

Chicken Stir-Fry with Brown Rice

1 chicken breast, cut

1 bell pepper, sliced 1 cup snap peas

1 carrot, sliced

1 tbsp soy sauce

1 tbsp sesame oil

1 cup cooked brown rice

Sauté chicken in sesame oil, add vegetables and soy
sauce, and stir-fry until cooked through. Serve over
brown rice.

Vegetarian Chili

1 can black beans, rinsed

1 can kidney beans, rinsed 1 can chopped tomatoes

1 onion, chopped 2 cloves garlic, minced

1 bell pepper, chopped 1 tbsp chile powder

1 tbsp olive oil

Salt and pepper to taste

Sauté onion, garlic, and bell pepper in olive oil, add beans, tomatoes, and spices. Simmer for 20 minutes.

Snack Options

Apple Slices with Almond Butter

1 apple, sliced 2 tbsp almond butter

A simple, nutritious snack that contains fiber and healthy fats.

Greek Yogurt with Honey and Walnuts

1 cup Greek yogurt

1 tbsp honey

2 tbsp chopped walnuts

Mix honey and walnuts into Greek yogurt for a protein-rich snack.

Carrot and Cucumber Sticks with Hummus

1 carrot, sliced

1 cucumber, sliced

1/4 cup hummus

A crunchy, fiber-rich snack with healthful fats from hummus.

Creating a balanced diet plan and building a menstrual health-friendly diet takes careful planning and selection of the proper foods. By concentrating on critical nutrients and adopting a range of complete, nutrient-dense foods, you can support overall health and decrease menstrual discomfort. These sample meal plans and dishes provide practical guidance for achieving a balanced and health-supportive diet.

Tips for Consistency

Consistency is the key to sustaining healthy eating habits. It's easy to get motivated and start a new diet or healthy eating plan, but it's much tougher to stick to it in the long run. However, with a few simple techniques and strategies, you can retain consistency and make healthy eating a habit.

First, it's necessary to create reasonable goals. Don't try to overhaul your diet at once. Instead, start with minor modifications that you can keep over time. For example, try adding a serving of fruits or vegetables to your meals each day, or substituting sugary drinks with water. As you get into the habit of making healthy choices, you can progressively make more major improvements.

Another key to consistency is preparing ahead. Take some time each week to plan out your meals for the next several days. Make grocery list and stick to it. Having healthy food on hand can help you resist the temptation of fast food or processed snacks. You can also prep meals in advance, such as preparing a huge batch of rice or roasting veggies, to make healthy eating easier and more convenient.

It's also crucial to listen to your body and be gentle to yourself. Remember that it's alright to indulge sometimes, and don't beat yourself up over a slip-up. Focus on getting back on track as soon as possible. Remember why you started making healthy changes in the first place, and let that drive you to keep going forward.

How to maintain healthy eating habits

Maintaining a healthy diet involves a combination of knowledge, planning, and self-awareness. By learning how different meals affect your body and mind, you can make informed decisions that promote your overall health and well-being. Here are some recommendations for keeping good eating habits:

Eat a variety of full, unprocessed foods, including fruits, vegetables, whole grains, lean meats, and healthy fats. Aim for a rainbow of colors on your plate to guarantee you're getting a range of nutrients.

Limit your intake of processed and packaged foods, which are generally high in added sugars, salt, and bad fats. Be especially aware of meals that are promoted as "healthy" but have hidden additives that can undermine your health goals.

Be cautious of portion sizes and restrict the amount of food you eat. Use a food scale or measuring cups to help you gauge your quantities, especially when eating out or consuming items that are high in calories.

Eat regularly to maintain constant energy levels and prevent overeating. Aim for three main meals and one or two snacks per day, depending on your unique needs.

Overcoming cravings and temptations

Overcoming cravings and temptations involves a combination of self-awareness, strategy, and support. Here are some techniques to help you combat cravings and stay on track:

Identify your triggers: Pay attention to when and where you tend to have cravings. Is it when you're stressed or bored? Do you crave particular foods when you're among certain people or in certain situations? Once you're aware of your triggers, you can design tactics to avoid or control them.

Find healthy alternatives: If you're craving something specific, try finding a healthier option. For example, if you're craving ice cream, try having a bowl of Greek yogurt with fresh berries instead.

Get enough sleep: Lack of sleep can boost the desire for unhealthy foods and make it tougher to keep to your healthy eating plan. Aim for 7-9 hours of sleep per night and focus on proper sleep hygiene.

Recall, adopting healthy eating habits takes time and effort. Don't be too hard on yourself if you mess up — instead, focus on getting back on track and celebrating your tiny triumphs along the road. With time and consistency, healthy eating will become second nature, and you'll be on your way to a healthier, happier self.

Chapter 11

Lifestyle Tips for Better Menstrual Health

Maintaining good menstruation health is important for general well-being. A healthy lifestyle can considerably relieve menstruation symptoms and increase the menstrual cycle's regularity and predictability. Here are several lifestyle tips to boost menstruation health:

Maintain a Balanced Diet

A balanced diet is essential for menstrual health. Consuming a range of foods helps balance hormones, lessen period pain, and maintain energy levels. Focus on including plenty of fruits, veggies, lean proteins, and whole grains in your diet. Omega-3 fatty acids, found in fish and flaxseeds, can help reduce inflammation and menstrual pain. Additionally, adding iron-rich foods like spinach, lentils, and red meat can counteract lethargy linked with menstruation.

Get Regular Sleep

Quality sleep is vital for hormonal balance. Aim for at least 7-9 hours of unbroken sleep each night. Establishing a consistent sleep routine, even on weekends, can help control your menstrual cycle. Creating a calming bedtime ritual, such as reading or having a warm bath, can enhance sleep quality and minimize period symptoms.

Limit Caffeine and Alcohol

Caffeine and alcohol can aggravate menstruation symptoms such as cramps, bloating, and breast tenderness. Reducing your intake of these chemicals, especially in the days preceding your period, can have a major effect. Instead, opt for herbal teas or water with a touch of lemon.

Complementary Practices

Complementary approaches can support and promote menstruation health alongside conventional methods. These techniques typically provide relief from menstruation discomfort and promote overall wellness.

Herbal Remedies

Various herbs have been traditionally used to treat menstruation discomfort. However, it is vital to contact with a healthcare provider before starting any herbal regimen.

Chasteberry: Often used to regulate hormones and alleviate symptoms of PMS, including breast discomfort, mood swings, and headaches.

Acupuncture

Acupuncture is a traditional Chinese medicinal treatment that includes inserting tiny needles into particular spots on the body. It is thought to restore equilibrium and flow of energy. Some research suggests that acupuncture can help reduce menstruation pain, control periods, and enhance overall reproductive health.

Aromatherapy

Aromatherapy uses essential oils to enhance physical and emotional well-being. Certain essential oils including lavender, clary sage, and rose can help ease period cramps and reduce stress. Using these oils in a diffuser, as a massage oil, or in a warm bath can give comfort.

Exercise and Physical Activity

Regular physical activity is vital for preserving menstrual health. Exercise helps balance hormones, lessen menstruation discomfort, and enhance mood.

Aerobic Exercise

Engaging in aerobic activities like walking, jogging, swimming, or cycling can enhance cardiovascular health and lower the severity of menstruation symptoms. Aim for at least 150 minutes of moderate aerobic exercise every week.

Strength Training

Strength training exercises help build muscle mass and support overall body strength. Implementing exercises like weight lifting, resistance band training, and body-weight exercises such as push-ups and squats. Strength training twice a week can help regulate menstruation discomfort and enhance overall health.

Yoga and Stretching

Yoga incorporates physical postures, breathing exercises, and meditation. It can considerably lessen menstruation discomfort, stress, and anxiety. Certain yoga poses, such as the child's pose, cat-cow, and supine twist, are particularly good for reducing menstrual cramps.

Pelvic Floor Exercises

Strengthening the pelvic floor muscles through exercises like Kegels can enhance menstrual health by strengthening pelvic support and reducing pain. These activities also enhance reproductive health and overall pelvic function.

Stress Management Techniques

Managing stress is crucial for maintaining hormonal balance and menstrual health. Chronic stress can increase menstruation symptoms and interrupt the menstrual cycle. Including stress management tactics into your routine might have a positive influence.

Mindfulness and Meditation

Practicing mindfulness and meditation helps calm the mind, reduce stress, and increase emotional well-being. Techniques such as deep breathing, progressive muscular relaxation, and guided imagery can be particularly useful.

Deep Breathing: Taking slow, deep breaths helps stimulate the parasympathetic nervous system, promoting calm. Practice deep breathing techniques for a few minutes each day to control stress.

Progressive Muscle Relaxation: This technique entails tensing and then relaxing each muscle group in the body. It helps alleviate bodily stress and promotes mental calm.

Guided Imagery: Visualizing serene and calming scenes helps relieve stress and increase emotional well-being. Use guided imagery recordings or develop your mental images.

Journaling

Writing out your thoughts and feelings can be a therapeutic method to manage stress. Journaling about your experiences, emotions, and menstrual symptoms can help you acquire insights into your health and uncover trends.

Time Management

Effective time management decreases stress by allowing you to prioritize chores and build a balanced schedule. Use tools like planners, to-do lists, and apps to arrange your time effectively. Ensure you allocate time for self-care and relaxation.

Social Support

Building a solid support network is vital for managing stress and preserving mental wellness. Surrounding yourself with supportive friends, family, and colleagues. Share your feelings and experiences with them, and seek support when needed.

The Role of Sleep in Menstrual Health

Sleep is a vital part of total health, strongly influencing physical, mental, and emotional well-being. Its significance extends to menstrual health, where it plays a key role in controlling hormonal balance, treating menstrual symptoms, and sustaining regular cycles.

Hormonal Balance

Adequate sleep is vital for maintaining hormonal balance. The body's endocrine system, responsible for hormone production and regulation, is very active during sleep. Key hormones like melatonin and cortisol, which control reproductive hormones, are regulated during sleep-wake cycles. Melatonin, produced in the pineal gland during sleep, has antioxidant qualities that protect ovarian follicles and maintain reproductive health. Cortisol, the stress hormone, is regulated throughout sleep, helping to maintain balanced levels that prevent hormonal abnormalities.

Menstrual Cycle Regularity

Sleep impacts the regularity of the menstrual cycle. Poor sleep patterns and inadequate sleep can impair the production of reproductive hormones such as estrogen and progesterone. Irregular sleep schedules can lead to irregular menstrual cycles, making it difficult to forecast periods and manage symptoms. Consistent, quality sleep encourages the regular release of these hormones, ensuring a more predictable menstrual cycle.

Managing Menstrual Symptoms

Adequate sleep is vital for managing menstruation symptoms. During sleep, the body conducts repair and restoration processes that minimize inflammation and pain. Lack of sleep can increase menstruation symptoms such as cramps, migraines, and mood swings. Quality sleep helps to ease these symptoms by allowing the body to recuperate and retain its natural equilibrium.

Emotional and Mental Health

Sleep has a huge impact on emotional and mental health, which in turn affects menstrual health. Poor sleep can lead to increased stress, worry, and sadness, all of which can exacerbate menstrual symptoms. Quality sleep boosts mood, reduces stress levels, and enhances emotional resilience. This pleasant mental state contributes to greater menstruation health and general well-being.

Immune System Support

Sleep boosts the immune system, which has a role in menstrual health. A healthy immune system helps the body control inflammation and infection, minimizing the likelihood of menstrual-related disorders such as infections or inflammatory illnesses. Adequate sleep ensures the immune system functions efficiently, offering additional support for menstrual health.

Natural Remedies and Supplements

Natural therapies and supplements might be effective in treating menstruation symptoms and maintaining overall menstrual health. While they should not replace medical advice or treatment, these options can provide additional support and relief.

Herbal Remedies

Herbal treatments have been used for generations to manage menstruation discomfort and boost reproductive health. Some commonly used herbs include:

Black Cohosh: Often used to control symptoms of menopause, black cohosh can also help ease menstrual cramps and regulate cycles. It works by mimicking the actions of estrogen in the body.

Essential Oils

Essential oils can provide relief from menstruation discomfort through aromatherapy and topical application. Some beneficial essential oils include:

Lavender: Known for its calming and relaxing characteristics, lavender oil can help alleviate menstruation pain and tension. Inhaling lavender oil or utilizing it in a massage oil might bring comfort.

Clary Sage: This essential oil has been proven to alleviate menstruation cramps and enhance mood. It can be used in a diffuser, as a massage oil, or added to a warm bath.

Peppermint: With its cooling and analgesic qualities, peppermint oil can help reduce headaches and muscle tension associated with menstruation. Applying diluted peppermint oil to the temples or abdomen can bring relief.

Rose: Rose oil has soothing and anti-inflammatory characteristics that can help ease menstruation discomfort and mental anguish. Using rose oil in aromatherapy or as a massage oil can be relaxing.

Dietary Supplements

Certain dietary supplements can improve menstrual health by supplying critical nutrients and lowering symptoms. Commonly recommended supplements include:

Magnesium: This element is vital for muscle relaxation and can help lessen menstrual cramps. It also helps emotional well-being by relieving symptoms of anxiety and despair. Food's rich in magnesium include leafy greens, nuts, seeds, and whole grains. Magnesium supplements can also be taken to ensure appropriate intake.

Vitamin B6: Vitamin B6 is vital for hormone regulation and can help minimize symptoms of PMS, such as mood swings and irritability. It also supports the development of neurotransmitters that influence mood. Food's rich in vitamin B6 include poultry, fish, bananas, and fortified cereals. Supplements might provide additional help.

Iron: Iron is needed during menstruation owing to blood loss. Ensuring appropriate iron intake can avoid anemia and sustain energy levels. Food's rich in iron include lean meats, beans, spinach, and fortified cereals. Iron supplements may be necessary for persons with low iron levels.

Lifestyle Modifications

In addition to natural therapies and vitamins, several lifestyle alterations can improve menstrual health and lessen symptoms.

Healthy Diet

A healthy diet rich in vital nutrients can drastically alter menstrual health. Consuming a range of fruits, vegetables, whole grains, lean proteins, and healthy fats ensures the body obtains the vitamins and minerals it needs to function efficiently.

Building a Support Network

Having a support network can bring emotional comfort and practical assistance during menstruation. Share your experiences and feelings with friends, family, or support groups. Seek expert support if needed to manage symptoms and enhance overall well-being.

Monitoring Symptoms

Keeping note of your menstrual cycle and symptoms can help you spot patterns and triggers. Use a period diary or mobile app to document your cycle, symptoms, and any lifestyle factors that may affect your menstrual health. This information can be beneficial when discussing your health with a healthcare provider.

Utilizing natural therapies, nutritional supplements, and lifestyle alterations can greatly enhance menstruation health and general well-being. By concentrating on a holistic strategy that includes appropriate sleep, stress management, and a balanced diet, you can effectively control menstruation symptoms and promote hormonal equilibrium. Always contact with a healthcare physician before starting any new regimen to ensure it is safe and appropriate for your unique needs.

Conclusion

Achieving and maintaining optimal health is a multidimensional task that involves a combination of dietary decisions, lifestyle improvements, and mindfulness activities. Menstrual health, in particular, benefits substantially from these holistic approaches. By concentrating on a balanced diet, sufficient hydration, regular physical activity, and stress management, individuals can dramatically enhance their overall well-being and menstrual health. This complete method not only alleviates symptoms but also promotes long-term health and vigor.

Recap Key Points

On the journey towards better menstrual health, several essential factors have emerged as fundamental. Understanding these ideas can aid in making educated decisions that support a healthier lifestyle.

Firstly, sleep has a critical function in regulating hormones and keeping a regular menstrual cycle. Adequate sleep encourages the generation of melatonin and cortisol, which are necessary for hormonal homeostasis. It also aids in regulating menstrual symptoms such as cramps, headaches, and mood swings by letting the body undergo the required repair and restoration processes.

Secondly, natural therapies and supplements can provide great relief from menstrual problems. Herbal treatments like chasteberry, ginger, turmeric, and black cohosh have been traditionally used to manage symptoms and support reproductive health. Essential oils such as lavender, clary sage, peppermint, and rose give additional advantages through aromatherapy and topical application. Dietary supplements include magnesium, vitamin B6, calcium, vitamin D, omega-3 fatty acids, and iron enhance overall menstrual health by supplying important nutrients and lowering discomfort.

Thirdly, lifestyle adjustments, including stress management strategies and a balanced diet, are necessary. Practices such as mindfulness, meditation, regular physical activity, and maintaining a support network can considerably reduce stress and promote

emotional well-being. A nutritious diet rich in key
nutrients and sufficient hydration further supports
menstrual health.

Summary of Foods to Avoid and Why

Dietary choices have a dramatic impact on menstrual
health. Certain meals can increase symptoms and alter
hormonal balance, making it crucial to understand which
foods to avoid and why.

Processed Foods: Processed foods often contain
additives, preservatives, unhealthy fats, and high
quantities of sodium. These can contribute to
inflammation, bloating, and hormone abnormalities.
Foods such as packaged snacks, fast food, and ready-
made meals should be limited in favor of complete,
nutrient-dense options.

High-Sugar Foods: Excessive sugar intake can lead to
insulin resistance and increased production of androgen
hormones, which can interrupt the menstrual cycle and
exacerbate symptoms like acne. Reducing the use of

sugary drinks, candy, and baked goods can assist preserve hormonal balance.

Refined Carbohydrates: Foods prepared with refined flour, such as white bread, spaghetti, and pastries, can induce fast spikes and decreases in blood sugar levels. These changes might influence energy levels and mood, leading to increased menstruation symptoms. Choosing whole grains instead can provide more consistent energy and improve overall wellness.

Dairy items: Some individuals may find that dairy items increase symptoms such as bloating, cramping, and acne. This may be related to the presence of hormones in dairy that might influence estrogen levels. Opting for plant-based dairy substitutes can help lessen these impacts.

Caffeine: High caffeine intake can contribute to increased anxiety, poor sleep, and worsening of menstruation symptoms such as breast tenderness and cramps. Limiting the usage of coffee, tea, and energy drinks can help lessen these effects.

Alcohol: Alcohol can interfere with sleep, hydration, and hormone control, leading to worsening menstruation symptoms and irregular cycles. Reducing alcohol intake or choosing non-alcoholic alternatives can have a good impact on menstrual health.

Salty Foods: High-sodium foods can lead to water retention and bloating, which can be particularly uncomfortable during menstruation. Reducing intake of salty snacks, processed foods, and restaurant meals can help reduce these symptoms.

Encourage Readers to Make Positive Changes

Making positive adjustments to improve menstruation health and general well-being is a journey that requires commitment, mindfulness, and support. While the work may seem onerous, starting with tiny, attainable actions can lead to tremendous long-term rewards.

Firstly, prioritize sleep. Establish a consistent sleep schedule, build a peaceful nighttime routine, and ensure your sleeping environment is favorable to slumber.

Quality sleep is important to hormone balance and general wellness.

Incorporate natural therapies and supplements into your regimen with assistance from a healthcare expert. Herbal medicines, essential oils, and dietary supplements can provide further support in controlling menstruation discomfort and promoting reproductive health.

Adopt lifestyle alterations that enhance stress management and emotional well-being. Practice mindfulness, participate in regular physical activity, and establish a support network. These behaviors not only promote menstruation health but also boost overall quality of life.

Focus on a balanced diet rich in key elements. Choose full, nutrient-dense foods over processed choices, avoid sugar and refined carbohydrates, and remain hydrated. Making conscious dietary choices can substantially improve menstrual health and alleviate symptoms.

Be proactive in tracking your menstrual cycle and symptoms. Use a menstruation diary or smartphone app to track patterns and identify triggers. This information can be beneficial when discussing your health with a healthcare provider.

Lastly, don't be scared to seek expert help. Consulting with healthcare providers, dietitians, and mental health professionals can provide helpful insights and personalized recommendations. They can help you design a thorough strategy that suits your particular needs and supports your journey toward better health.

In conclusion, obtaining better menstrual health is a comprehensive approach that entails making informed nutritional choices, implementing supportive lifestyle activities, and seeking expert help when needed. By prioritizing sleep, adopting natural remedies and supplements, reducing stress, and focusing on a balanced diet, you can greatly enhance your menstrual health and general well-being. Embrace these beneficial improvements with patience and determination, and remember that little, regular measures can lead to substantial long-term advantages